BSAVA

MANUAL OF CANINE BEHAVIOUR

Valerie O'Farrell

PhD Chartered Psychologist

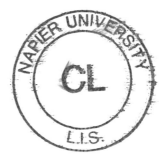

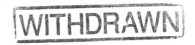

A Company Limited by Guarantee in England.
Registered Company No. 2837793.
Registered as a Charity.

Typeset by Michael Gorton Design,
Worthing, West Sussex.
Printed by Grafos S.A., Barcelona, Spain.

The publisher cannot take any responsibility
for information provided on dosages and methods
of application of drugs mentioned in this publication.
Details of this kind must be verified by individual users
in the appropriate literature.

First Published 1986
Second Edition 1992
Reprinted 1996, 1998

ISBN 0 905214 17 X

THE AUTHOR

Valerie O'Farrell graduated from Oxford University in 1963 in Psychology, Philosophy and Physiology. She trained in Clinical Psychology at the Institute of Psychiatry, London and obtained a Ph.D. in Abnormal Psychology on the subject of obsessional rituals. She also trained in psychotherapy at the Tavistock Clinic, London. She held the posts of Lecturer in the Department of Psychology, University College, London and in the Department of Psychiatry, Edinburgh University. She became interested in the application of psychology to the understanding of problem behaviour in pets and, since 1982, has been attached as a Postdoctoral Fellow to the Small Animal Practice Teaching Unit of the Royal (Dick) School of Veterinary Studies in Edinburgh. She is engaged in research into dog behaviour problems and provides a consultancy service for the owners of small animals with behavioural problems.

PREFACE TO
THE SECOND EDITION

Since I wrote the first edition of the Manual of Canine Behaviour six years ago, the topic of dog behaviour problems has become more widely accepted as a proper object of scientific study. Many more papers on the subject have been published. My own further clinical experience and informal discussion with colleagues have also caused me to alter my approach to some problems. I have tried to incorporate into the second edition the new insights and information now available.

I should also like to thank the following for their help:

Fellow animal behaviourists David Appleby, Judith Blackshaw, John Fisher, Don McKeown, Peter Neville and John Rogerson; Harvey Locke and Colin Price of the BSAVA publications committee; Jane Gough for her speedy and efficient typing.

VALERIE O'FARRELL
1992

ACKNOWLEDGEMENTS

I should like to offer my thanks to the following:

to Dr. Peter Darke and my colleagues at the Royal (Dick) School of Veterinary Studies for their help and support; to BP Nutrition who funded some of my research; to the B.S.A.V.A. who have made this publication possible; to Mr. Colin Price, the Chairman of the Publications Committee, for his efficiency, patience and good sense; to Dr. Simon Carlyle for his help in grappling with the mysteries of word processing; to Mr. Henry Carter, Mr. Andrew Edney and Dr. Bruce Fogle for reading and commenting on drafts of the typescript; to Michael Gorton Design for the printing and cover design; to family and friends for their help and encouragement; particularly Mrs. Gillian Jordan, my father Professor Nigel Walker and my husband Paul.

Lastly, I would like to thank the referring veterinary surgeons and their clients and patients, without whom this book could not have been written.

V.O'F.

FOREWORD

The rapidly expanding science of Animal Behaviour has yielded much knowledge of clinical relevance to practising veterinary surgeons. There is now sufficient information on the normal and abnormal behaviour of dogs for a publication on this subject and the BSAVA has commissioned this work, the first of its kind in the United Kingdom, to assist veterinary surgeons in this increasingly important area of small animal practice.

Dr. Valerie O'Farrell has collated the information available and drawn on her own clinical experience gained at the Small Animal Practice Teaching Unit of the Royal (Dick) School of Veterinary Studies. The text is divided into two sections: the first providing the theoretical background to the second, clinical section. This should equip the practising veterinary surgeon with sufficient knowledge to approach cases of normal canine behaviour with more confidence, allowing him to formulate treatment regimes where appropriate and assisting him in the selection of those cases which require referral for specialist advice.

COLIN PRICE
Chairman, Publications Committee
1986

CONTENTS

PART ONE
BASIC PSYCHOLOGICAL PROCESSES

Chapter One

      Incidence of problem behaviour in dogs
      History of canine psychology
      Learning theory
      Ethology
      Developmental psychology
      Relevance of human clinical psychology

Chapter Two

      Nature of thought processes
      Intelligence
      Language
      Moral sense
      Rule following

Chapter Three

      Classical conditioning   Shaping
      Instrumental learning   Secondary reinforcement
      Reinforcement   Punishment
      Extinction   Shock collars
      Stimulus generalisation

Chapter Four

      Social interaction among wolves   Hunting and feeding
      Dominance hierarchy   Play
      Territory   Breeding
      Owner – dog relationships
      Expression and establishment of dominance
      Dominance and the veterinary consultation
      Dominance and dogs in the same household

Chapter Five

      How phobias are learned and unlearned
      Manifestations of high arousal
      Displacement activities
      Conflict
      Personality differences

Chapter Six

      First three weeks
      Socialisation period
      Development after fourteen weeks

CONTENTS

PART TWO
TREATMENT OF SPECIFIC DISORDERS

PART ONE

BASIC PSYCHOLOGICAL PROCESSES

INTRODUCTION

Chapter One _____

**Incidence of problem behaviour in dogs;
history of canine psychology; learning theory; ethology;
developmental psychology;
relevance of human clinical psychology.**

The British are supposed to be a nation of dog lovers and the dog is one of Britain's most popular pets. It is easy to understand why; dogs are by nature social animals which readily form close attachments to human beings. A dog can be your friend in a real sense; a goldfish can be a friend only in your imagination.

But there is a price to be paid for this friendship. Because dogs, and usually their owners, expect to live on intimate terms together, there is room for misunderstanding and friction.

A comparison with cats is illuminating. Cats, although possessing a cognitive capacity similar to dogs, do not have the same inborn need for social relations. They usually occupy a quite different position in the household: they live their own lives and are not required to conform to the owner's wishes. For example, cat owners usually do not expect automatic affection from their pet; they are honoured if it pays them attention. They do not expect automatic obedience either. They will normally take care to remove a tasty piece of fish from the kitchen table, rather than leave the cat alone with it, and will usually accept the consequences philosophically if they forget.

By contrast, a dog's constant affection is often taken for granted. **Its owners often regard the dog as an almost human member of the family (Wilbur, 1976) and expect it to assume social responsibilities to match this position.** Many dog owners would be outraged if the dog helped itself to food left on the table.

It is not really surprising, therefore, that the incidence of 'problem' behaviour in dogs is fairly high. A survey of 50 unselected dog owners attending the Small Animal Practice Teaching Unit of the Royal (Dick) School of Veterinary Studies for veterinary treatment revealed that 10 of their dogs did things which caused them definite inconvenience: aggression towards themselves or visitors for example. Another 30 had less serious behaviour problems such as behaving excitably with visitors or having a fear of the vacuum cleaner. Only 10 owners considered they had a perfectly behaved dog. American surveys (Houpt, 1976; Wilbur, 1976; Voith, 1984) of much larger numbers of owners (350-1500) have found a range of 25-42% of owners considering their dog's behaviour to be a problem. It seems likely that the differences in these percentages can be explained by differences in the definition of problem behaviour.

At its most serious, problem behaviour can be life-threatening for the dog, in the sense that it cannot be tolerated and euthanasia is the only option. In addition, many behaviour problems which the owner chooses to tolerate significantly impair the quality of life of dog and/or owner. It is not unknown for families to cease having visitors to the house because of an excitable or aggressive dog or to give up going out together because of a dog which barks or is destructive in their absence.

Such tolerance may often seem surprising to an outsider, but there are various reasons why owners continue to keep a dog under such circumstances. Voith (1981), interviewing the owners of dogs and cats with behavioural problems, found that the reason most commonly given was that the owner was attached to the animal. It must be borne in mind that for the majority of problem dogs the undesirable behaviour forms only a small part of their repertoire; most of the time they are affectionate and lovable pets. An owner of a hyperactive dog which barked constantly described a common predicament: 'I often think I can't stand it any longer, but then I imagine setting off with him to the vet for the fatal injection and I know I just couldn't do it'.

Another factor which stops many owners from ridding themselves of a problem dog is a feeling of responsibility for its behaviour. The view that 'there are no bad dogs, only bad owners' is fairly widespread and owners of problem dogs have often taken this maxim to heart. They have searched their past and present behaviour towards the dog for faults and, of course, have found things to feel guilty about. Friends and relatives have usually suggested a few more; in our society, like criticising other people's child-rearing methods, finding fault with how other people handle their dogs is a popular pastime. One result of this tendency to blame the owners for the dog's behaviour is often that owners feel morally obliged to continue living with a problem they feel they have produced in the first place. Many of these owners struggle on unaided; some seek help at obedience classes or from dog trainers. Only a small proportion seek help from veterinary surgeons.

This is not surprising, as it is only in the last ten years that veterinary surgeons have had any professional expertise to offer on the subject of behavioural problems. Although many of them were able to offer advice which turned out in some instances to be helpful, this was simply because they had seen and handled many dogs. A sensible dog breeder or handler could have come to the same conclusions; they were not based, as are a veterinary surgeon's other professional opinions, on a scientific body of knowledge.

The veterinary surgeon who wants to include treatment of behaviour problems in the services he offers may need to inform clients of this, rather than wait for them to raise the subject themselves. One way of doing this might be to enquire routinely about behaviour as part of general health checks.

HISTORY OF CANINE ABNORMAL PSYCHOLOGY

It was nearly 20 years ago (e.g. Tuber *et al,* 1974) that it began to be realised that theory and experimental work from various aspects of psychology could be used to devise methods of treating behaviour disorders in animals. Many of the theories were formulated and the experiments carried out over 20 years before, but their relevance for pet owners had not been realised.

Much of the most useful work came from **'learning theory'**. This is really a collection of different models, all experimentally based, whose aim is to explain how organisms, including human beings, acquire behaviour patterns which are not instinctive. The psychologists who worked in this area in the 1940s and 1950s were keen to establish psychology as a science as respectable as the physical sciences. They felt it to be of paramount importance that they study only 'hard' data: events which could be observed and measured. They considered thought processes and ideas difficult if not impossible to measure and they confined themselves to studying behaviour. When this perspective is adopted, experiments with animals have several advantages over human experiments; the behaviour of animals is, by and large, less complex; it is easier to control all aspects of an animal's life. So many thousands of animals of various species were subjected to a variety of learning experiences, the best known of which were, perhaps, Pavlov's dogs, pigeons in Skinner boxes and rats in mazes.

> **In terms of the distress caused to the animals involved, some of these experiments, including some described in this book, were ethically dubious, to say the least. It would be foolish, however, not to take note of the findings which emerged from them, especially as they can now benefit living animals.**

The applications of this body of theory based on animal work were, to begin with, mainly in the human field and in the 1950s it was proposed that it had relevance to the treatment of some psychiatric disorders. It was postulated that if some psychiatric patients could learn not to engage in their abnormal behaviour then they would, *ipso facto,* be cured. If an agoraphobic could be taught to go out or a transvestite could learn not to put on women's clothes, they would cease to be ill; to cure the symptom was to cure the disorder. It was found that behaviour therapy, the collection of methods based on this theory, was extremely successful with some disorders which up to then had not responded to psychiatric treatment. It was perhaps at its most successful in dealing with 'monosymptomatic' phobias, (i.e. a fear of some fairly definite or circumscribed situation, such as spiders or flying in an aeroplane), in patients of otherwise normal personality. This success led in the 1960s to a wave of enthusiasm for behaviour therapy, which began to die down in the 1970s when therapists discovered that patients' mental processes, their capacity to reflect on their actions or use one thing as a symbol for another, often made a nonsense of dealing only with their observable actions. Thus an agoraphobic patient might turn out to be less afraid of streets and open spaces than of the loneliness and lack of structure which they represented. In the same way a transvestite's fascination for women's clothes might prove to be the most obvious manifestation of an abnormality in many other aspects of his relationships with other people.

At the same time, independently, animal behaviourists were realising the potential application of behaviour therapy to the species on which it was originally developed. Not surprisingly it has proved more successful in this field than in the human field.

> **An animal's cognitive processes are less complex than a person's; it does not brood over the past, worry about the future or, most importantly, it does not think symbolically.**

It is influenced to a much greater extent by the present situation. Thus if a dog has a fear of something, say gunfire, or shows aberrant sexual behaviour, say mounting the sofa cushions, it is much safer than in the case of a human being to assume that this fear or this sexual behaviour is simply a learnt response to the stimulus in question and is not a sign of another more pervasive fear or indicates a more far-reaching disorder of personality.

The other branch of psychology which has been found relevant to the treatment of animal behaviour disorders is *ethology,* the study of instinctive, as opposed to learned, behaviour. This field of study was developed in the 1940s by such workers as Lorenz and Tinbergen. Schenkel (1947) initiated the study of the nearest wild relative of the dog, the wolf, using an ethological frame of reference. But again it was only in the 1970s that the relevance of this work for pet owners was appreciated.

Developmental psychology, the study of the way animals and humans grow and change mentally and behaviourally during their life-span, has also proved useful. The most important workers in this area were Scott & Fuller in the 1940s, followed by Fox in the 1950s. They studied the psychological development of puppies and the ways in which different environments could affect it. Their findings do not provide such useful tools as learning theory or ethology for correcting problem behaviour, but they do help to provide explanations as to why particular dogs are susceptible to behaviour disorders; they are particularly relevant for people such as dog breeders, who are in a position to prevent behaviour problems.

There is one discipline whose relevance has become evident more recently: **human clinical psychology.** With the growth of interest in the relationship between owners and their pets (sometimes referred to as the 'human/companion animal bond') it has been pointed out by psychiatrists and psychologists such as Beck & Katcher (1983) that pets can benefit people in more subtle ways than merely encouraging them to take exercise or giving them an 'interest'. They can provide special kinds of relationship which fulfil psychological needs that may not be met in other ways; a dog is often more than just a dog to its owner. Not only is it usually regarded as a family member, but it may also be something on which affection which has no other outlet can be lavished, or it may provide an acceptable outlet for aggression. There is now some evidence (O'Farrell, 1992) that this kind of psychological use of a dog can have an effect on the development of behaviour problems in the dog and therefore is a dimension which should be borne in mind when treating behavioural problems.

The aim of this book is to provide the veterinary surgeon with enough knowledge of the various areas of psychology and their application to treatment to enable him to treat at least some behaviour problems himself. As with physical disorders, the veterinary surgeon will encounter, from time to time, serious or complicated cases which need to be referred to a specialist. But for every case like that there will be several cases which he could treat himself, if properly informed.

> **Behaviour problems cannot be treated by the blind application of mechanical procedures; they require an appreciation of the unique combination of causes operating in each individual case. This book therefore does not consist of a collection of 'treatment recipes'. It consists of two sections, one theoretical and one practical. The theoretical section provides an overview of the various aspects of psychology relevant to the understanding and treatment of behaviour problems. The practical section deals with the kinds of problem commonly encountered, the factors which are often involved in their causation and possible approaches to treatment. It also deals with the prevention of behaviour problems.**

COGNITIVE PROCESSES: THINKING AND LEARNING

Chapter Two _____

**Nature of thought processes; intelligence;
language; moral sense; rule following.**

2.1. NATURE OF THOUGHT PROCESSES

**When a dog is a much loved member of the household, affectionate and
devoted to its owners, it is easy to fall into the habit of assuming that
it thinks like a human being.**

The human mind is the kind we are most familiar with and when we try to read sense into the action of another creature it is natural to use this model. But this assumption is often mistaken; it can give rise to a tangle of misunderstandings which lead to problems or make existing problems worse.

Psychologists, on the other hand, over the last half century have tended to go to the other extreme and attribute no thought processes to animals. Because of their concern to deal in hard, observable data, their experiments measured only behaviour (for example how many times a rat turned left or right in a maze or how much food it ate). The most extreme form of this approach was that of B.F. Skinner who considered it was not profitable to speculate at all about what goes on inside an organism. He regarded it simply as a 'black box', measured only input and output and attempted to calculate equations connecting the two. He and his colleagues were remarkably successful in this endeavour and hard-core learning theory now consists of a number of laws relating input (stimulus) to output (response), which allow the optimum conditions for learning to be calculated. Although from a modern perspective this undertaking seems misguidedly mechanistic, within their own limits these 'laws' have proved extremely useful in human education; the teaching of the handicapped in particular has been revolutionised. They are also very relevant to the training of animals, including dogs; following a Skinnerian model when trying to teach a dog to do (or not do) something results in efficient learning. The next chapter is devoted to explaining the rules of this model in more detail.

Because this model has been so successful, the question of what goes on inside the animal's mind has been rather neglected. It has been assumed that, below the level of primates, an animal responds automatically, without conscious reflection, on the basis of associative learning; that its responses are habitual, built up from past experience and that its consciousness is rather like that of a car driver who drives without thinking and arrives at his destination without any idea of how he got there. To put it another way, it was assumed that Pavlov's dogs, which learned to salivate at the sound of a bell when the bell had been frequently paired with food, did so automatically and unconsciously without formulating any expectations or theories, such as 'The bell means food'. On the other hand, recent research in the learning theory tradition has produced findings which can only be explained by postulating that animals do after all have expectations and formulate theories (Mackintosh, 1974). There is also plenty of other evidence that animals and, more specifically, dogs do more than just automatically associate stimuli and response. One task which requires more than just this automatic association is the 'delayed response', where the subject is shown a reward being hidden under one of two or more identical cups or similar receptacles. After a certain delay the animal is allowed to choose one of the receptacles. Beritoff (1971) has shown that dogs can perform this task successfully with an intervening delay of up to half an hour and even after having gone to sleep during the interval. It has also been shown that wolves have 'mental maps' of their territory. They can find their way from one place to another by the shortest route, not necessarily a route which they have ever taken before.

Dog owners and dog handlers are usually able to recall many incidents illustrating the same point. The wisest conclusion seems to be that

although the model of associative learning is a useful one and will help one predict and control a dog's behaviour in most situations, it should always be borne in mind that it is an oversimplification and does not do justice to the complexities of a dog's mind.

2.2. INTELLIGENCE

The question of whether dogs vary in intelligence is an interesting one which can cause feelings to run high among owners and breeders. Scott & Fuller (1965) carried out various tests, which might be described as tests of mental ability, on puppies of various breeds. They found that different breeds were better at different tasks. For instance, beagles were the best at solving a spatial problem whereas basenjis were the best at a task which involved manipulating objects. They concluded that there was no one kind of ability which could be called intelligence in dogs, because each task required specific abilities. Although this is a tactful conclusion and one which was in keeping with the behaviourist ethos of the time, it is not a legitimate one. Human intelligence is customarily measured by a battery of tests. Performance on each of these may be affected by different specific factors such as level of anxiety or manual dexterity, but performance on all of them is also determined by a general factor of intelligence. This can be estimated by taking scores on all these tests into account. It seems likely that in a similar way it would be possible to devise a battery of tests which would measure canine intelligence and that it would be possible meaningfully to categorise dogs as more or less intelligent. As was mentioned at the beginning of this chapter, however, **it is probably more important when diagnosing and treating behaviour problems to be aware of the limitations rather than the extent of a dog's intelligence.**

2.3. LANGUAGE

However clever some dogs may be, it is certain that there are some mental feats involving symbolisation or high levels of abstraction which no dog can perform. For example, a dog cannot understand language in the ordinary sense of the term. Although it can learn to associate a word such as 'walkies' with a certain idea or expectation, it can never acquire any notion of grammar or syntax; it can never develop a notion that the same words differently combined can convey different meanings. For instance, a dog may learn what 'Sit' means and what 'Dinner' means but learning these two commands would never enable it to make sense of the command 'Sit in your dinner'. **A dog can therefore never understand more than a tiny fraction of what its owner says to him. The reason why owners feel understood by their dogs is that dogs are extremely good at reading non-verbal communications: expressions, gestures and tone of voice;** (see Chapter 4) and can correctly predict an owner's actions or interpret his wishes from these cues.

Related to this is the fact that, although dogs obviously can form expectations about the future and have memories about the past, it is impossible to communicate with them in any complex way about past and future. Human beings are helped by language to move back and forward in time, but language is not available to dogs. This is relevant to problem behaviour which occurs in the owner's absence, such as food stealing, destructive chewing etc. There is no point in an owner saying before he goes "Don't you dare touch those sausages", nor is there any point in punishing the dog when he returns and finds the sausages eaten. In either case the owner's actions are too far separated in time from the misdeed to have any effect upon it.

2.4. MORAL SENSE

Also important where behaviour problems are concerned is the fact that **a dog cannot be said to have a moral sense: it cannot tell 'right' from 'wrong'.** Problems which arise over dogs' behaviour are frequently made worse because the owner is not only inconvenienced by what the dog has done but feels outraged and let down by the dog's action. He often feels confirmed in his opinion that the dog knows it is doing wrong by the dog's submissive or fearful demeanour afterwards. **The owner often interprets this behaviour as guilt, but it is in fact simple fear of punishment, untinged by moral overtones.** This kind of misunderstanding commonly complicates problems of destructiveness in the owner's absence. The owner comes back to find the carpet chewed and the dog crouching in a submissive apprehensive posture or slinking away into a corner. As well as being upset about the carpet, the owner often thinks 'He knew it was wrong to do that; see how guilty he looks. He must have done it to get attention or get back at me for going out'. Depending on the owner's temperament, he may punish the dog to show it it can't get away with that sort of thing or lavish more attention upon it to make it feel less neglected. Either of these manoeuvres is likely to make the situation worse rather than better (see Chapter 10.7)

2.5. RULE FOLLOWING

A related point is that a dog is incapable of following a rule in the way we understand the term. It may reliably walk to heel on the pavement because it has formed the habit of so doing, but it has not understood that it must not run in the road. This means that although ninety-nine times out of a hundred it may stay on the pavement out of harm's way, on the hundredth time it may, because of extreme provocation such as the sight of a cat on the other side, run into the road. The fact that dogs never come to understand a rule in the same way as we do is reflected in the way that the learning process proceeds. Much of our own learning takes place by being told rules by other people ('Stand in that queue if you want to buy stamps') or by working them out for ourselves ('Thursday must be early closing day because these shops are shut'). Once we have understood the rule we can move at once from a situation of uncertainty to a situation where we get it right every time. Thus, once we have grasped which is the stamp queue, we stand in it every time we go to the Post Office to buy stamps. But a dog's learning is not characterised by this sudden change; from 'getting it wrong' most of the time, it progresses gradually, getting it right more and more of the time, until it gets it right most of the time.

This point is relevant to the training of dogs and to the prevention of behaviour problems. **An owner cannot assume that once a dog has learnt a habit such as staying in the garden or walking on the pavement it has learnt it for all time; he should always bear in mind that an exceptional circumstance might tempt the dog to lapse.**

In human learning it is sometimes said that we learn most from our mistakes. This is because mistakes help us to discover a rule or principle which we can use subsequently. The same is not true for learning in dogs. **The more often a dog does the right thing, the higher the probability that it will do so in the future. Situations where the dog might be tempted to do the wrong thing are to be avoided.**

FURTHER READING

WALKER, S. (1983). Animal Thought. Routledge and Kegan Paul, London.

COGNITIVE PROCESSES: LEARNING THEORY

Chapter Three

Classical conditioning; instrumental learning; reinforcement; extinction; stimulus generalisation; shaping; secondary reinforcement; punishment; shock collars.

Although learning theory, as we have seen, does not do full justice to a dog's cognitive abilities, it is the most powerful model available at the moment for predicting and changing a dog's behaviour. It is extremely useful in explaining and treating behaviour problems and this chapter is devoted to setting it out in some detail. 'Learning theory' is really a collection of slightly different theories evolved by different workers. What follows is an exposition of the common ground of these theories which would be accepted by most psychologists.

Animals can learn new behaviour in two ways: via instrumental learning or classical conditioning. Instrumental learning occurs when an animal learns to perform a voluntary response in order to get a reward of some kind (as when a rat learns to press a lever in order to get a food pellet) or avoid punishment (as when a guinea pig learns to jump over a barrier into another part of the cage to avoid a shock).

CLASSICAL CONDITIONING

3.1. Classical conditioning differs from instrumental learning in that (a) it concerns involuntary or reflex responses rather than voluntary movements; and (b) no reward is involved. If a stimulus (technically known as the unconditioned stimulus) which naturally or instinctively provokes a reflex response (unconditioned response) is repeatedly paired with a previously neutral stimulus (conditioned response) then eventually the neutral stimulus on its own will provoke the reflex response (conditioned response). The best known example of this phenomenon is its earliest demonstration by Pavlov, using dogs. The unconditioned stimulus used was food, the unconditioned response being salivation. At the same time as food was presented to the dogs, a bell was rung (conditioned stimulus). Eventually the dogs salivated when they heard the bell on its own.

The same process can be applied to responses of more interest to owners than salivation; these are mostly responses mediated by the autonomic nervous system. Sexual behaviour is one example. Breeders make use of the phenomenon of conditioning to ensure reliable performance in their stud dogs; normally the bitches visit the dog and the stage is set by the breeder in a stereotyped way. The mating takes place in the same room, perhaps even on the same piece of old carpet. Eventually the sexual response of the dog becomes conditioned to the breeder's preparations, the room etc. and does not depend so much on the attractions of the particular bitch.

The sexual response of the pet dog can also become conditioned in the same way to seemingly bizarre objects such as a rug or a teddy bear. (Of course it can also become conditioned to human beings but this is probably a more complex process which is discussed in Chapter 11.5). The relevance of this observation is that this kind of activity does not mean that the dog is 'over-sexed'; if the object to which the response has become conditioned is removed, the behaviour may well disappear. How the sexual response became conditioned to the particular object in the first place may often be obscure; a likely explanation in many cases is that it arose during puberty, when the dog's sexual responses were relatively disorganised and not yet focused on their proper object.

House training

Classical conditioning is also involved in responses normally of great interest to owners: urination and defaecation. The unconditioned stimuli for these responses are internal bodily sensations and environmental stimuli such as the scent of previous urination. House training is the process of conditioning these responses to some environmental stimuli and not to others. Most owners are content if the responses are conditioned to out-of-doors stimuli and not to in-the-house stimuli, but it is possible to condition the responses to much more specific stimuli, such as the gutter or a piece of grass. **Because this learning is based on classical conditioning rather than on instrumental learning (see Section 3.2) an external reward is not essential.** The owner's task during house training is to arrange that as far as possible the unconditioned stimuli coincide with the desired conditioned stimuli; i.e. that the dog is taken outside after meals, after sleep and when it starts sniffing around for scent marks. The owner does not need to reward successes or punish failures. House-training can be a tiresome business anyway, involving standing around in cold winds at unsocial hours, waiting for the dog to perform. It can become even more trying, however, if the owner mistakenly sees the process as a battle of wills. Some owners find the whole business much easier if they realise that their own relationship to the dog is not central to it.

There is another important class of response which can be classically conditioned: **emotional responses.** These are discussed in Chapter 5.

3.2. INSTRUMENTAL LEARNING

> **The basic principle of instrumental learning is that if an action (response) performed in a certain situation (stimulus) is followed by a reward (reinforcement) then when that situation occurs again the probability of the action being performed is increased.**

This basic principle in itself is neither new nor startling. It is the principle used in standard methods of dog training, where for example the dog is told to sit (stimulus) and when it sits (response) it is praised (reinforcement). It is the elaborations and refinements of this principle which are of more interest. Those most relevant to behaviour problems are as follows:

GENERAL

It is an important point that this principle refers merely to the coming together of three events: stimulus, response and reinforcement. It states that whenever three events of this kind occur together, the animal's subsequent behaviour will be altered. The animal does not have to be in a particular 'learning' frame of mind, nor does there have to be a teacher. Moreover when the learning is arranged by someone, the role of this teacher is not to convey to the animal a rule of behaviour; his role is merely to arrange for stimulus, response and reinforcement to occur in such a way that learning takes place. All this has several implications:

a. **Dogs go on learning even when no-one intends to teach them anything.**

Much problem behaviour is a result of this accidental learning (see 3.3c for examples).

b. **Obedience classes.**

Owners may prefer to train their dogs in the context of a training class because they (the owners) have become accustomed from childhood to doing their learning in special situations called 'classes'. For the dog, any situation is a potential learning situation. The ordinary domestic environment has much to recommend it (see Chapter 12.13).

c. A teacher of a class of human beings often has to be a showman, holding the attention of the audience, dominating and manipulating them, in order to hold their attention and impress upon them the importance of what he is trying to convey. Although a satisfactory relationship with a dog certainly involves dominating it (see Chapter 4.6), **an owner cannot teach a dog anything simply by dominating it.** The successful trainer of a dog is not a dominating showman, but an unobtrusive stage-manager arranging for the appropriate stimuli and rewards to occur at the right time. When a dog does not appear to be learning what is intended, the owner may become angry and repeat his commands in a louder and fiercer voice, as if to compel the dog to do what he wants. This is useless; the owner needs to detach himself from the situation and work out why the dog is not learning.

d. **Forced training.**

When teaching a particular response to a particular stimulus, arranging that the animal performs the required response can be a problem. How do you reward a dog for lying down on command when it shows no inclination to lie down in the first place? Many training manuals advocate forcing the dog into the required posture to 'show' it what is required. But the aim of training is not to teach a rule of behaviour or explain to the dog what to do, but to arrange for stimulus, response and reinforcement to occur together. It is, therefore, far more effective to reward the dog when it actively takes up the required posture of its own free will than if it is passively forced into it. To teach a dog to perform on command an action which it frequently performs spontaneously, it is usually sufficient to wait until the dog starts to perform it and then quickly say the word of command. If the owner says 'Sit' every time he sees his puppy sitting down and then immediately rewards it, it will soon sit on command. For an action which is performed less frequently, it is often necessary to use some ingenuity to put the dog in a situation where it will choose to perform it. For example, one method of teaching a dog to lie down is to put a tit-bit on the floor between the dog's front paws, with a cupped hand over it, in such a position that the dog has to crouch down in order to try to get it. As the dog goes down the owner says 'Down' and removes his hand, so that the dog is rewarded with the tit-bit; it is also praised verbally. When this response is established, the hand is still placed on the floor but the tit-bit is gradually omitted on an increasing number of trials, the dog being rewarded by praise alone (see 3.7). Eventually the dog will go down on command without the hand being placed on the floor at all.

It should have become evident from the foregoing discussion and examples that **training a dog is a slower business, making more demands on patience and ingenuity, than many people expect.** If this is true of training in standard obedience drill, it is even more true of the correction of learned problem behaviour. It is important that the veterinary practitioner emphasises this to owners seeking treatment of problem behaviour, as many expect a quick and easy solution via medication or training carried out by some other person. **If the owner is not able or willing to devote some time to curing the problem, it might be better not to attempt treatment.**

3.3. NATURE OF REINFORCEMENT

What kind of events are reinforcing (rewarding) to a dog? In terms of the theory, the definition has a certain circularity in that reinforcing events are those which promote learning. In practice it is fairly easy to tell what things are rewarding for a dog; they are the things which he anticipates with obvious eagerness or makes some effort to obtain. So food, praise and petting are rewarding to most dogs and these are the reinforcements most commonly used in dog training. However, there is a much wider range of experiences which many dogs will also find rewarding: for example, going out into the garden, having a ball thrown, looking out of the window or receiving attention from the owner. Dogs differ in their enjoyments, but most owners know what their own dogs find rewarding. These points are important to bear in mind because:

a.   **It is better when training a dog to use a variety of reinforcements.**
This will make it more likely that the response will generalise to other situations where a particular reward is not available.

b.   Some dog training manuals give the impression that some kinds of reward (e.g. food) are somehow morally undesirable. This seems to be based on the view that if a dog does something in order to get praise from its owner, the proper relationship between dog and owner is maintained but if it does something in order to get a tit-bit, the relationship is put on an undesirable footing because the owner is 'bribing' the dog or the dog is 'blackmailing' the owner. However, as Chapter 2 should have made clear, teaching a dog does not have a moral dimension. Also, as was pointed out in 3.2c, the training of a dog is a separate matter from becoming dominant over it. **Thus it makes sense in any given situation to use the most effective rewards,** whether they be food, praise, petting or some other experience. Praise has advantages as a reward in certain situations. It can be delivered at a distance and takes no time to absorb, which does not apply to food. On the other hand, for many dogs a delicious tit-bit, such as a piece of cheese, can provide an incentive which no amount of praise and petting can match. It is a matter of matching the reinforcement to the training situation.

c.   **In looking for explanations of problem behaviour which seems learned rather than instinctive, it is often worth searching for the hidden reward.**
For example, dogs which bark frantically in the car are often rewarded by the car continuing on its journey, passing interesting sights and perhaps eventually arriving at one of the most exciting of destinations: the start of a walk. Social reinforcement from the owner can be the hidden reward in many situations. A dog which has periods of annoying hyperactivity in the house, barking or pestering people for attention, often has owners who pay it more attention when it is restless than when it is quiet. Even when this attention takes the form of being cross with the dog, it can act as a reinforcement. Sometimes the crossness is not forceful enough to be perceived as such by the dog (we have all seen owners who say 'Bad dog' in such a mild way that the dog is not upset at all).

3.4. TIMING OF REINFORCEMENT

The timing of a reward is crucial: it must be delivered at the same time as the response to be reinforced, or immediately afterwards; a delay of even one second can weaken the effect. Longer delays can mean that a response other than the one intended is reinforced. Thus a chocolate drop given to a dog at the end of a training session, 'because he has been such a good boy', has no beneficial effect. It probably has no adverse effect either (other than reinforcing the behaviour of hanging around in the hope of receiving chocolate drops) but there are situations where a reward, wrongly timed, can have the opposite effect to that intended. It is worth investigating this possibility in cases where owners seem to be treating a learned behaviour problem correctly, but no progress is being made. For instance, an owner may be attempting to cure his dog's habit of begging for food at human meal times by training it to sit in its basket. He may do this by telling the dog to go to its basket, then calling it to come to him and rewarding it with a tit-bit. This is more likely to reinforce the dog's action of coming to the owner (which is exactly what he wanted to discourage).

3.5. INTENSITY OF REINFORCEMENT

It would seem at first sight that the more pleasant a reward is and the greater the incentive it provides, the more effective it will be. Experimental work has shown, however, that too high a level of motivation and arousal can have a disruptive effect on performance and that the optimum level of motivation decreases as the complexity of the task increases. This generalisation is known as the Yerkes-Dodson Law. So, in an emergency while driving the car, terror will make us apply the brake extremely quickly and effectively, but extreme nervousness in an examination can make us do less well than we might otherwise have done. When applied to learning in dogs, this means that **when an owner is trying to evoke a simple response, such as coming when called, an extremely attractive reward, such as a delicious tit-bit, should be used. On the other hand, when the response is more complex or calls for calmness and self-control (for example sitting still when visitors arrive) a very attractive reward may have a counter-productive effect because it may increase the dog's excitement.** Mild praise is often an appropriate reward in these circumstances.

3.6. EXTINCTION

Extinction is the technical term for what happens when a response is unlearned. If a learned response is never reinforced it will eventually be extinguished, although responses which have been previously reinforced only on some occasions will take longer to extinguish (see 3.7). **Ensuring that a response is never rewarded is the safest, most reliable way of eliminating it from an animal's repertoire.** Where feasible, it is always preferable to punishment (see 3.11). For example, an owner who wants to stop a dog begging for food should just ignore it, rather than shout at it or smack it. **When a response which has previously been reinforced is suddenly not reinforced, that response is initially performed more frequently, before its frequency starts to decline.** This phenomenon has discouraged many owners who have tried to extinguish annoying habits in their dogs by withdrawing the reinforcement of their attention. They may say 'We tried ignoring him when he pestered us, but he just got worse'. The answer to this objection of course is that persistence will eventually lead to a decline in the behaviour.

3.7. SCHEDULES OF REINFORCEMENT

When an animal is being taught a response, it will learn most quickly if the response is reinforced every time it occurs. When teaching a puppy to sit, it is best to give it a reward every time it sits. However, a response which has been reinforced every time is relatively easy to extinguish; if the puppy has come to expect a reward every time it sits, when the reward ceases to appear it will soon stop sitting. Once a response is established, the frequency of reinforcement should be gradually reduced. **The responses which are most resistant to extinction are those which are reinforced at irregular intervals.** This often applies to learned problem behaviour and makes it particularly difficult to extinguish. For instance the owners of a dog which pesters them for food at human meal times may have consistently given it tit-bits at the table when it was a puppy because it looked so sweet and appealing. The response of begging for food would be quickly learned under these circumstances. As the dog grew larger, its begging behaviour might well have become more of a nuisance. At this stage arguments might break out in the family about giving the dog tit-bits; the more hard-hearted members might have stopped feeding it, while the soft-hearted members continued. This would have the effect of gradually reducing the reinforcement. In the end, everyone might become tired of the dog's behaviour. By this time, however, it would have become accustomed to reinforcement at variable intervals. Although the family might manage totally to ignore it for a while, someone eventually gives the dog something 'to keep it quiet' or even just speaks to it and tells it to go away (social reinforcement). Because of the reinforcement history of the behaviour, this is enough to perpetuate it.

3.8. STIMULUS GENERALISATION

This is the process whereby a response learned to a particular stimulus is likely also to be performed in the presence of similar stimuli.

A dog which has developed a fear of the sound of gunfire may also panic at the sound of any loud noise. In the same way, a dog which has developed the habit of barking when the bell rings, because it has learned to associate this sound with the arrival of visitors, may start to bark at other similar sounds, such as the telephone ringing or even ice-cream van chimes. As well as being involved in the development of many behaviour problems, this process of stimulus generalisation can also be useful in their cure. A dog which has learnt to bark at men calling at the house (e.g. postmen, milkmen) can be successfully treated if it can be taught not to bark at a few examples of the genre. Thus, if it can be taught to sit quietly while the milkman and the postman call, it will probably be calmer when the man calls to read the gas meter or when the window-cleaners arrive.

3.9 SHAPING

This is a method of teaching complex responses which are not already in the animal's repertoire, by reinforcing successive approximations to the desired response.

This is how animal trainers get their animals to do things they would be unlikely to do naturally, such as jumping through burning hoops or riding bicycles. Using the same methods, it is possible for owners to teach their dogs to do clever things around the house, for instance to open doors by manipulating the door handle. To achieve this, the dog might be rewarded for going to the door on command; then it would not be rewarded until it put its paws on the door; then it would have to put its paws higher and higher on the door before it received a reward; after that it would only be rewarded when it put its paws on the door handle; it would then be rewarded only if it pressed down on the door handle; finally it would be rewarded only when it pressed the handle and the door opened.

Most people do not want to teach their dog to do that sort of thing but there are 'tricks' which are more useful, if less spectacular. One is sitting quietly in a designated place (e.g. basket). To the owner of an excitable dog it may seem impossible that it could acquire this habit, because it never does anything remotely approaching this. However, it may well be possible to teach the dog this by means of shaping. For example, the dog is first of all rewarded for going to its basket, then for sitting there with the owner beside him. It is then required to sit there for gradually increasing lengths of time with the owner still beside him. After that, the owner may gradually move increasing distances away from the dog, coming back to reward it. Finally the dog is only rewarded when the owner has been out of sight and returned after increasing lengths of time.

3.10. SECONDARY REINFORCEMENT

Some events can act as reinforcers, not because they are intrinsically rewarding, but because of their association with intrinsically rewarding events. In a classic experiment, Wolfe (1936), showed that chimpanzees would perform tasks, such as pulling a heavy weight, if rewarded with poker-chips. They had learned earlier that these poker-chips would deliver raisins if posted in a vending machine. In the same way, police dogs searching for drugs are immediately rewarded for a find by giving them a graspable object, such as a piece of stick. This object has become rewarding for the dog because it has been previously associated with play and attention from the handler. An owner can make a toy into a secondary reinforcer for his dog in a similar way. All other toys are removed and, for the dog, taking the chosen toy in its mouth is made a pre-condition of all the nice things in its life: being fed, getting attention from the owner, etc. The toy can then be employed in the treatment of a range of bahaviour problems. It can be used as a focus of distraction/response substitution (see Chapter 8.8). It can be used as an anxiety reducer in systematic desensitization (see Chapter 10.1) and Chapter 8.8).

For most dogs, interaction with the owners is intrinsically rewarding and therefore praise is a primary reinforcer. Its value as a reward can be increased, however, by making it a secondary reinforcer also. This can be done by regularly pairing praise with tit-bits and physical contact.

Similarly, the punishing or aversive quality of some stimuli can be enhanced by pairing them with an unpleasant event (see section 3.11).

3.11. PUNISHMENT

Punishment is the most over-used technique in dog training.

For many owners, it is the method they first resort to when attempting to stop undesirable behaviour. The reason for its popularity may be its immediate benefits to the owner. If an owner comes downstairs in the morning to find the dog has defaecated on the carpet, it is hard for him to set about cleaning up the mess without addressing a cross word to the dog. A dog that stands watching, wagging its tail, with a puzzled but tolerant look on its face seems to add insult to injury. A dog cowering in the corner, having been smacked and shouted at seems much more appropriate. The owner's feelings have been relieved; he also feels he has done something to prevent the same thing from occurring again.

The underlying assumption that punishment has the opposite effect to reward is wrong. The opposite of reward is absence of reward; if a response is not reinforced, it will eventually be extinguished.

Sometimes an owner also seems to feel that the whole sequence of wrong action followed by punishment is beneficial, helping the dog to learn. This may be true for people, but it is not true for dogs (see 2.5).

Punishment is sometimes spectacularly successful in changing undesirable behaviour, but there are various possible pitfalls:

a. To stand any chance of being effective, punishment must be delivered within one second of the undesirable behaviour. There is, therefore, no point in taking a puppy to a puddle on the floor made half an hour previously and smacking it, or in shouting at a dog when the chewed remains of a slipper are discovered.

b. Even when delivered at the right time, there is a danger that the dog will associate the aversive stimulus with the wrong aspect of the situation. A common example of this kind of misunderstanding is a dog which apparently cannot be house-trained. Whenever the owner discovers the dog urinating in the house, he smacks it; when he thinks the dog needs to urinate, he takes it into the garden: it never urinates there, but when the owner gives up and brings it indoors, it immediately sneaks away into another room and urinates on the floor. This is because it has learnt to associate punishment not with urinating indoors, but with urinating in the presence of the owner.

c. The intensity of the aversive stimulus must be exactly right. If it is too strong, it may provoke fear or aggression. This is particularly undesirable if the punishment is perceived as coming from the owner. If the punishment is too weak, it will be ineffective.

d. If punishment is repeated, the dog is likely to become habituated to it. This means that it is difficult to find the right strength of an aversive stimulus by gradually increasing it, because at the same time the dog is habituating to it. It also means that even if a stimulus is effective in stopping the undesirable behaviour the first time, it may become ineffective on subsequent occasions.

e. Because of their past experience of punishment and because of their temperaments, individual dogs vary in their reactions to the same punishing stimulus: what has no effect on one may frighten another severely.

f. The more motivated the dog is to perform an action, the greater the intensity of punishment required to stop it.

g. Punishment tends to increase anxiety. Therefore, if the behaviour is motivated by anxiety in the first place (e.g. destructiveness in the owner's absence; see Chapter 10.7), punishment will make it worse.

h. After punishment, the undesirable response is much more likely to recur if an alternative response is not encouraged and rewarded.

From the foregoing, it can be seen that if punishment works, it works quickly: this explains the dramatic accounts of successful punishment (e.g. dogs permanently cured of food stealing by having a tablecloth pulled from under them). What people tend to keep quiet about are all the occasions when punishment was unsuccessful. **Behaviour modification which relies on rewards, extinction, distraction and response substitution takes longer, but is more reliable. Where it is possible to use these methods they are, therefore, preferable to punishment.**

It can also be seen that punishment is much more likely to work when the dog's motivation to perform the undesirable behaviour is comparatively low: a comparatively mild aversive stimulus is effective and does not run the risk of provoking fear or aggression. Owners correct most undesirable behaviour in this way by themselves (for instance by saying ''No'' in a sharp tone of voice). The problems for which expert help is sought are normally those which have not responded to punishment because the dog's motivation is too high. Owners are often advised by another owner to try a specific punishment which worked for his dog (e.g. hitting its nose with a rolled up newspaper when it pulls on the lead), but this is unlikely to be a correct level of punishment for a different dog. In addition, as mentioned in (f.) above, if the behaviour is motivated by anxiety, any punishment will make it worse.

However, if there is no alternative to punishment, its effectiveness will be maximised if these provisos are borne in mind:

a. The punishing stimulus is more appropriately viewed as a distracting stimulus: its aim is not to upset the dog or give it an unpleasant experience, but to disrupt the undesirable behaviour and divert the dog's attention from it.

b. Sometimes calling the dog's name is enough to achieve this aim of distraction. If not, a startling or novel stimulus is often effective, e.g. rape alarm, training disks (see f. below), water pistol, tin can with pebbles thrown or rattled.

c. In most sequences of highly motivated behaviour, there is usually a moment at the beginning of the sequence where motivation is comparatively low and the dog can be distracted comparatively easily. For example, for a dog which has developed a habit of catching letters as they come through the door and chewing them, this moment might be when the postman's steps are heard approaching the house. (When the owner is fortunate enough to foresee a provocative situation before it even arises — if, for example, he sees the postman approaching the house before the dog hears him he should intervene at this point).

d. Punishments which seem unconnected with the owner are preferable. They make it more likely that the dog will refrain from the undesirable behaviour even in the owner's absence. They also avoid the risk of arousing negative emotions towards the owner. When the owner has delivered a 'remote' punishment (e.g. a thrown object), he should not look cross with the dog. Instead, he should call the dog and reward it for coming to him: this provides an appropriate alternative response to the undesirable behaviour.

e. The most aversive feature of many punishing stimuli seems to be that they are unusual and unexpected, disrupting the normally predictable flow of events. This is why 'all-purpose' startling stimuli soon become ineffective: their aversive power depends on their novelty. But it also means that thwarting the dog suddenly and unexpectedly in its purpose can be aversive in itself. Thus, if a front door is unexpectedly shut in a dog's face as it runs out, or it is suddenly checked on an extending lead, it may be less eager to run out again.

f. **Pre-training**

Just as rewards such as praise can be made more rewarding for the dog if it is pre-trained to regard them as secondary as well as primary reinforcers, so stimuli can be made more aversive by pre-training. This seems to be the principle underlying the effectiveness of devices such as training disks (see Appendix). These disks consist of several metal circles threaded on a ribbon: they make a high pitched metallic sound when thrown onto a hard surface, such as the floor. Their success seems to depend on a pre-training schedule where the noise of the disks is immediately followed by a frustrating event, such as removing a tit-bit which the dog is about to eat. Dogs which initially do not react to the sound will often, after a few repetitions of the sequence, start to behave as if it were markedly aversive. The same pre-training can be undertaken for other stimuli, such as the sound of a bunch of keys being thrown or even a word spoken in a distinctive tone of voice. The stimulus must be one which does not occur in the normal course of events or it will either lose its aversive meaning or make the dog extremely anxious. For the same reason, it should not be employed routinely to stop the dog doing anything the owner does not like, but only for the treatment of a behavioural problem which is resistant to other methods.

g. After the undesirable behaviour has been successfully stopped by punishment or distraction, the dog should always be provided with another response which is intrinsically rewarding or is rewarded by the owner. Thus an owner might stop his dog chasing a cat in the garden by throwing a tin can which lands beside it with a clatter. He then immediately calls the dog to him and rewards it for coming or throws a ball for it to chase.

3.12. SHOCK COLLARS

Shock collars have aroused some controversy. They usually work by means of a battery and circuitry incorporated into a collar worn in the normal way. The collar is normally capable of delivering a shock to the dog when activated at a distance by a radio signal; sometimes a device is included which activates the shock when the dog barks. Often the intensity of the shock can be set at different levels. On the face of it, the collar has the following advantages:

a. It is capable of administering a stimulus unpleasant enough to disrupt most behaviour.

b. It is not obviously connected with the owner.

c. The remote control type can be operated at a distance, so that a dog's behaviour can be controlled even when it is out of physical reach of its owner. The type which is activated by barking works of course even in the owner's absence.

On the other hand, it also has the following disadvantages:

a. Although, in theory, in the case of the variable intensity types, it is possible to deliver a punishing stimulus just strong enough to stop the undesirable behaviour and no more, it would require careful adjustment and testing to ensure this. It seems very likely, especially if the collar were used by the general public, that traumatic levels of shock would be delivered. Apart from ethical considerations, this could have a counter-productive effect of increasing the dog's general level of anxiety or excitement.

b.   The collars activated by barking have particular disadvantages. Where the dog is barking out of excitement, punishment is in any case not an appropriate treatment. There is also a risk of the shock mechanism being activated by stimuli other than the one intended (e.g. other dogs barking, or loud noises). In these circumstances, the dog would receive shocks it could not avoid, which is an efficient method of producing a neurotic disorder (see Chapter 5). In addition, because they are designed to operate unsupervised in the owner's absence, there is a risk of even more unpleasant situations arising. For example, the dog might never learn not to bark to avoid the shock but might yelp and bark whenever it was shocked, thus setting up a vicious circle from which it could not escape.

It is, therefore, inadvisable and even unethical to operate these collars except under expert supervision.

Where expert supervision is available, the use of the radio-controlled collar might be appropriate under the following conditions:

a.   the behaviour disorder is severely anti-social and cannot be treated without the use of punishment;

b.   the behaviour is an isolated disorder in an otherwise normal dog; more particularly the dog is not abnormally aggressive or neurotic.

c.   the undesirable behaviour is not motivated by anxiety.

A behaviour disorder which often meets these criteria is sheep-worrying and it has been successfully treated using a shock collar.

FURTHER READING

BORCHELT, P. and VOITH, V. L. (1985). Punishment. The Compendium on Continuing Education for the Practising Veterinarian. **7**, 780-788.

SAUTER, F. J. and GLOVER, J. A. (1978). Behaviour, Development and Training of the Dog. Chapters 5, 6 and 7. Arco Publishing Company, New York.

SOCIAL BEHAVIOUR

Chapter Four _____

Social interaction among wolves: dominance hierarchy; territory; hunting and feeding; play; breeding; owner – dog relationships: expression and establishment of dominance; dominance and the veterinary consultation; dominance and dogs in the same household.

Part of the reason for the dog's popularity as a pet is its sociable nature. The dog is a pack animal, born with the potential ability to recognise and perform a whole repertoire of social responses. It is important to bear in mind that, to a large extent, a dog's social repertoire is innate; what is learned is:

a.   the species towards which the dog directs its social behaviour; **dogs which have contact with human beings during the first twelve weeks of life regard them as members of their own species (i.e., as potential social objects);**

b.   the part of the social repertoire which is used; for example, all dogs have the potential for both dominant and submissive behaviour, but have to learn to whom it is appropriate to show which behaviour.

Although the 'social map' every dog is born with is similar enough to the human view of social relationships to enable communication to take place and relationships to be formed between the two species, the differences are great enough to leave room for misunderstandings to occur. The social nature of the dog which can give so much pleasure can also give rise to problems.

SOCIAL INTERACTION AMONG WOLVES

The easiest way to understand a dog's ethology in general, and social behaviour in particular, is to study wolves. There are two reasons for this. Firstly, most dogs live in a social world which includes human beings as important members. To try to make sense of such interactions is like trying to understand a play in which some actors do not know their parts properly. Secondly, in the process of domestication of the dog, certain elements of behaviour have become distorted so that it is hard to appreciate their significance or how they fit into the whole pattern. For instance, wolf bitches which have cubs in the process of being weaned will regurgitate food for them. Some dog bitches do this, but in such a disorganised way, vomiting in the puppies' absence or eating the regurgitated food themselves, that the behaviour appears purposeless. In addition, some aspects of the behaviour of some breeds is hard to interpret because of its neoteny; that is, as a result of selective breeding, some breeds tend still to show as adults behaviour which is more characteristic of the immature wolf. The tendency of some breeds to be friendly towards strangers is one example.

Because of their timidity and nomadic habits, it is hard to study wolves in their completely wild state. However, workers such as Zimen (1981) have achieved a satisfactory compromise by keeping wolves in a semi-wild state in large enclosures. A summary of the relevant parts of their observations is set out below, but in order to appreciate the richness and complexity of the wolves' interactions it is necessary to read an original account such as Zimen's. It is clear, however, from such accounts that even years of painstaking observation of this kind has not enabled us to understand the wolves' social system fully; what follows is a summary of the best established facts.

4.1. DOMINANCE HIERARCHY

A wolf pack consists of an extended family of both sexes. A wolf will live all its life in this pack, unless it breaks away to form a new one. The pack moves around, hunts and feeds together. Breeding occurs between pairs within the pack, which then co-operates to rear the cubs. A great deal of the wolf's social behaviour seems aimed at reinforcing this social cohesion. Wolves often urinate in turn on the same spot; they also regularly gather in a group and howl. In addition, several times a day (e.g. after sleep), wolves will greet each other muzzle to muzzle and sniff each other's ano-genital regions. These behaviours seem to have no function other than promoting group solidarity and ensuring that each pack member can easily recognise the others.

The concept of the dominance hierarchy applies to wolf social behaviour, but is more complex than is commonly supposed. Males and females tend to have separate hierarchies. Dominant animals tend to instigate activities and have prior claim over resources such as food. They tend to be older and heavier animals. The dominance hierarchy is not a rigid one, however (Lockwood, 1979); the social structure of a wolf pack is not like an army, where an individual has a fixed rank. It is more like a human family; in a family, different members tend to take charge, depending on the activity. Also, individual wolves differ in the extent to which they are preoccupied with dominance.

There are several implications for dog behaviour.

a. **Scott and Fuller (1965) have shown that dogs which have had even the most minimal contact with human beings before the age of 12 – 14 weeks will regard their owners as belonging to their pack; some of them will, therefore, form dominant/subordinate relationships with their owners. With these dogs, if the owner does not intentionally make clear where he stands in the hierarchy, the dog makes what sense it can out of the owner's unintentional cues and jumps to its own conclusions.**

b. A dog may take the dominant role in some situations and not in others. For example, it is not unknown for dogs which perform well in obedience trials to behave dominantly towards their owners at home.

c. Not all dogs are preoccupied with dominance. Only owners of dominant dogs need to be concerned about maintaining dominant status over their dogs (see 4.7).

4.2. TERRITORY

For most of the year, wolves move about a fairly large area, covering perhaps twenty square miles. On the whole, this territory is visited by only one pack and is staked out, particularly at its boundaries, by urine and faeces marking. The intensity of this marking increases if the pack discovers evidence of intrusion by another pack. During the summer months, if there are cubs being reared, the pack does not move around so much. The mother of the cubs settles in a smaller area, with perhaps several dens in it and the rest of the pack make forays from and return to this focal point. This 'home area' is defended more fiercely than is the wider territory. Higher ranking wolves in the pack are engaged more actively in defence and do more urine marking, as if part of the responsibilities of their high status were to guard the pack's territory against intrusion.

For many dogs, their house, garden and often the car constitute the 'home' area. The degree of interest shown in defending this area may be related to the dog's perception of his dominance status. If a dog's tendency to guard its territory becomes problematic, it may be necessary to alter its dominance status in the household (see Chapter 9.2). Similarly frequency of urine marking may be related to dominance status; where this behaviour becomes a problem (e.g. if it occurs in the house) reducing the dog's dominance may be helpful. A dog may perceive its home territory as including areas away from home where it is habitually exercised, such as the local park. If inclined to inter-dog aggression, it may be more aggressive to dogs encountered there than in a strange place.

4.3. HUNTING AND FEEDING

The ability of wolves to hunt in an organised group greatly increases the size of the game they can hunt; wolf packs in Canada can bring down adult moose. The efficiency of this hunting group is also increased by the tendency of its members to follow a leader. The survival value of a dominance hierarchy is very evident here. In feeding, an order of precedence is also evident.

For many pet dogs, access to food may also be important in determining how they perceive their dominance status (see Case Example 8.1). One way of reducing dominance, or preventing it from developing, is to ensure that the dog

(a)   never sees itself as successfully demanding food from its owner and

(b)   is often required to be obedient or submissive to the owner in order to be fed (see Chapter 9.2).

(c)   sees its food being prepared before the owners' meal, but is not fed until after their meal.

4.4. PLAY

Although play is a characteristic activity of the young of many species, wolves are unusual in that the adults often play with one another. Play can be distinguished from serious activity by one or more of the following characteristics:

a.   two wolves or dogs playing will change roles frequently, e.g. the aggressor will become the victim;

b.   parts of a behaviour sequence will be performed in isolation or juxtaposed with behaviour from another sequence; thus two wolves or dogs playing together might show sexual behaviour, aggressive behaviour and prey-catching behaviour towards each other, all in the space of a few minutes;

c.   there are postures which are characteristic of play: the 'play bow' (see Figure 1) which is an invitation to play is the most obvious but there is a certain lightness and springiness which, when it accompanies otherwise serious actions, also denotes playfulness.

Figure 1.

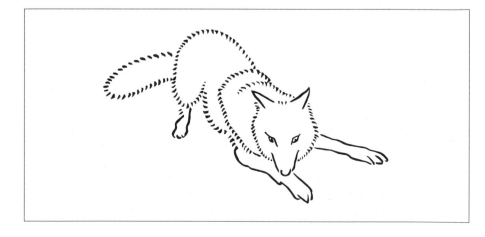

For young animals, play has the underlying serious purpose of providing practice in behaviour which will be required in later life. For example, in play fighting, the acceptable limits of biting may be learned. For adult wolves, play seems to have various underlying serious social purposes. This aspect of social interaction is as yet not adequately understood; but it seems that adult wolves use play in similar subtle ways to adult human beings. Although on occasions they seem to be simply enjoying themselves, they may also use play to advance their social status, to test out a prospective adversary, or to deflect aggression.

The implications for a dog owner are:

a. he may be falsely reassured by the playful nature of his dog's aggression. **A great deal of playful aggression directed towards another dog or towards a human being may signal serious aggression in the future.** In the case of two dogs living together, a certain amount of playful aggression is normal, but if it suddenly escalates it may be a sign that a struggle for dominance is starting. The same applies to play aggression towards people and as it is always desirable that the dog be firmly in the subordinate position in these relationships, **owners should not fight in play with dogs which are inclined to dominance.**

b. Some games, such as tug-of-war, which do not involve fighting are, nevertheless, 'dominance' games. With dominant dogs, these too should be avoided.

c. When a young puppy bites his owner in play, the owner should squeal as if in pain and immediately stop the game. This mimics the normal response of another puppy and will teach it to inhibit play biting.

4.5. BREEDING

Wolves do not become sexually mature until they are around two years old. Although puberty for dogs is normally much earlier (six to twelve months), personality changes can take place at two years as well, presumably mediated by further hormonal changes; for example, male dogs may make a bid for dominance at this time.

Female wolves come into oestrus only once a year around February. Fighting in the pack tends to increase in the weeks before the females' oestrus, as the necessity to establish a dominance hierarchy becomes more urgent. The more subordinate females may not even show behavioural signs of oestrus. Mating usually takes place between more dominant animals, although individual idiosyncratic preferences also play a part in partner choice. A pair bond formed between a dominant and a relatively subordinate individual may result in the elevation of the status of the subordinate one.

For the purposes of selective breeding, as many animals as possible need to be capable of and willing to mate with any partner the breeder chooses. Breeders have, therefore, selected against the kind of choosiness shown in a wolf pack. However, some dogs and bitches do still show individual preferences. Also, the failure of a bitch to come into full oestrus and behave responsively towards the male may on occasion be related to her subordinate position in a hierarchy of bitches.

There is little doubt that dogs can distinguish human genders and that they can form relationships with people which involve sexual drives and behaviour. This can affect how they perceive their own dominance status. If a dog or bitch forms a close attachment to an opposite sex human being of high status in the family this can raise its own perceived dominance status. For example, it is fairly common in problems of dominance aggression to find, if the dog is male, that it has formed a close attachment to the wife in the family, with or without overt sexual behaviour. In these cases, the situation often improves if the person involved ignores the dog so that it has to look to the rest of the family for attention and social interaction.

Women seem to find it more difficult than men to establish dominance over a male dog. This may be because his natural inclination is to seek to form a pair bond with a female, dominance hierarchy relationships usually being formed between animals of the same sex. It is significant that women who are successful at dominating male dogs (e.g. breeders of large aggressive breeds) often do it by pretending to be men (i.e., by assuming a gruff voice and male gestures). In addition, some women may find the behaviour required to establish dominance (see 4.8) at odds with their conventional role of nurturance and compliance.

4.6. EXPRESSION OF DOMINANT/SUBORDINATE RELATIONSHIPS BY DOGS

Wolves use body language to establish and express their dominant and subordinate relationships to one another. Dogs use similar body postures, though long coat, dropped ears or absence of tail may make these harder to interpret.

SUBMISSION is expressed in any of the following ways:

a.   The gaze is averted.

b.   Active submission: the dog crouches down, ears back, tail lowered (see Figure 2).

c.   Passive submission: the dog rolls on its side with one leg in the air exposing the inguinal region in a characteristic posture (see Figure 3).

DOMINANCE is expressed by:

a.   Meeting the owner's gaze.

b.   Standing with ears forward, tail up, the hair on the neck may be raised, the lips forward in a characteristic expression (see Figure 4).

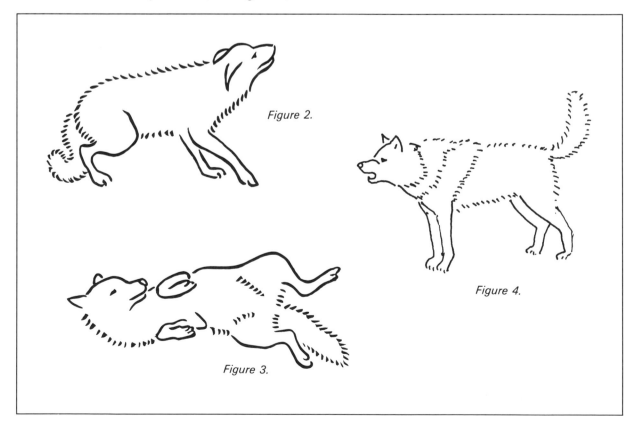

Figure 2.

Figure 4.

Figure 3.

c. A dog can express its dominance over another by standing over it, typically at right angles, with its forepaws on the other's back. Puppies playing often take up this position. By analogy, a dog may feel more dominant over its owner if it is allowed to put its paws on his shoulders or, in the case of a smaller dog, put its head and paws on his lap or curl round his neck or shoulders.

Any situation in which the relative heights of owner and dog is reduced tends to make the dog feel more dominant. For example, allowing a dog to sleep on the owner's bed can enhance its dominance.

d. Apart from its body language, a dominant dog tends to behave in characteristic ways:

   i. It may become increasingly difficult to move it from its resting place; for example, it may be reluctant to leave a chair if the owner wants to sit there.

   ii. It may be unwilling to give up things it has in its mouth and it may be possessive about food.

   iii. It may be slow to obey commands.

   iv. It may object to being groomed or excessively patted or cuddled.

   v. Most importantly, it has been shown that, in general, in species such as monkeys and wolves which form dominance hierarchies, the dominant animals initiate the most social interactions and respond to the fewest.

Where a dog is showing dominance aggression, it is common to find that in the household it initiates a high proportion of activities it participates in. Typically, it does not hang around its owner all the time pestering for attention; it will only approach its owner from time to time and they usually respond to this greeting. It may also let its owners know when it is time for its meals and walks or when it wants to be let into the garden. Even if it is not showing dominance aggression, a dog which behaves in this way probably sees itself as dominant and there is, therefore, a risk that it may become aggressive in the future (see Chapter 9.2).

4.7. AGGRESSION AND DOMINANCE

Aggression by the dog should not be regarded as an expression of dominance, similar to the behaviours outlined above (Abrantes, 1987). Aggression may, indeed, be shown by dogs in a dominant role, but also by dogs in a subordinate role. In fact, it is a sign that the normal conventions of behaviour have broken down. A subordinate dog may bite when frightened or cornered (see Chapter 9.2). A dog which perceives itself as dominant in a relationship may attack if it feels its dominant body signals have not been appropriately responded to by a perceived subordinate.

Some dogs seem to dispense with the social conventions and resort to aggression more readily than others. There are also breed differences. Bradshaw and Nott (1992) found that in litters of Cavalier King Charles spaniel puppies, dominance relationships were communicated by signals so subtle that they could only be detected by means of slow motion video replay. In litters of French bulldogs, on the other hand, the dominance structure was obvious and fights broke out frequently.

4.8. EXPRESSION OF DOMINANCE / SUBMISSION TOWARDS THE DOG

A human being can express dominance or submission towards a dog in the following ways:

a. Meeting the dog's gaze signals dominance. Averting the gaze signals submission. If the dog growls or threatens, averting the gaze is the first avoiding action to take: it may prevent attack.

b. Being taller than the dog signals dominance; being lower signals submission. This is why, when attempting to make friends with a strange dog, one should crouch down to its level.

c. The dominance effect of standing over a dog is augmented by patting or grooming it; this is why, if a dog bites its owner, this commonly happens when the owner is handling it in some way. Many owners feel they can empathise with a dog which turns nasty while it is being groomed ('he doesn't like having his hair brushed') but feel outraged if it snaps at them when they are patting it ('I was only trying to be friendly').

d. Claiming a resource, such as food, resting place, or territory.

e. Giving the dog a command.

f. **Ignoring all the dog's social initiatives, paying attention to it only when it obeys a command, or otherwise behaves in a submissive way, is an extremely effective way of asserting dominance.** It also involves no risk of provoking aggression from the dog. This is the method of choice for owners of dominant dogs (see Chapter 9.2: treatment of dominance aggression).

4.9. DOMINANCE AND THE VETERINARY CONSULTATION

A veterinary surgeon's attitude and behaviour towards his client and his patient may sometimes be determined by incorrect assumptions about dominance:

a. It is not uncommon that a dog which cannot be controlled by the owner is easily handled by the veterinary surgeon. This is usually due to the fact that the veterinary practitioner is a relative stranger to the dog and therefore not established in a subordinate relationship.

b. Some veterinary surgeons assume that the best way to ensure that a dog will comply with veterinary procedures and refrain from biting is to 'dominate' it. They may do this with actions which do indeed indicate dominance to the dog (e.g. standing over it, meeting its gaze, getting hold of it); they may also try to stop any untoward behaviour by speaking sharply to the dog or even hitting it. Aggression of this kind is completely inappropriate (see 4.7) and is likely to provoke fear and /or defensive aggression in the dog. Actions which really do signal dominance are usually best avoided also, as they encourage the dog to construe the situation in those terms. It is usually advisable to behave in a non-threatening manner.

4.10. DOMINANCE AND DOGS IN THE SAME HOUSEHOLD

Dogs in the same household usually manage peacefully to work out and maintain a dominance hierarchy. Sometimes, however, fights break out. As explained in 4.7, this indicates that the social conventions are not working properly. **It is a mistake to assume that if left to themselves, fighting dogs will settle their disputes without serious injury.**

Owners should be especially concerned if

i. either dog is of an aggressive breed;

ii. there is a marked disparity in the sizes of the two dogs;

iii. either dog has an early history of poor socialisation to other dogs, which might make it less able to understand the other's body language.

Clear differences in status and fierce fights over dominance occur mainly among high-status wolves; life at the top is competitive. Similarly, if two dogs in a household are fighting in earnest, a contributory factor may be that they both perceive themselves to be fairly dominant in the household; if the owner becomes more dominant over both dogs, this may ease the problem.

When there is serious fighting between two high-status wolves, there is likely to be more fighting in the rest of the pack as well; it is as if the uncertainty about leadership unsettles everyone and those with ambition lower down the scale seize the opportunity to improve their own status. Similarly, in cases of dominance aggression in dogs, it may emerge that the aggression developed during a period of family disagreement in the household.

FURTHER READING

ZIMEN, E. (1981). The Wolf. London: Souvenir Press.

STRESS, ANXIETY AND AROUSAL

Chapter Five

**How phobias are learned and unlearned;
manifestations of high arousal; displacement activities;
conflict; personality differences.**

In the modern world our attention is constantly being drawn to the pervasive effect of stress and anxiety on human functioning, both mental and physical. It is not so often realised that these factors can also operate in a wide range of canine disorders. It is outside the scope of this book to discuss the physical disorders which might on occasion be considered as psychosomatic, but in many behaviour disorders anxiety can also play a role which is not immediately obvious.

In the previous three chapters, the differences between human and canine psychology have been emphasised, because in the realms of cognitive functioning and social behaviour owners tend to assume too much similarity between the two species. On the other hand, where anxiety or other states of general excitability are concerned, the similarity may be greater than is superficially apparent; the behavioural manifestations of such states may differ in human beings and in dogs, but the underlying psychological processes are often similar. This behavioural divergence (and, therefore, the risk of misinterpreting the dog's actions) is greater in the case of activities motivated by a general high level of arousal of anxiety (see 5.4) than it is in the case of specific fears or phobias (5:1-3).

FEARS AND PHOBIAS

5.1. FEAR

Fear is usually defined as an intensely unpleasant experience, the person who is afraid showing at least one of the following characteristics:

a. **Flight or avoidance behaviour.** The person tries to escape from or avoid the feared situation.

b. **Extreme alertness plus autonomic activity.** A person who is afraid may be over-alert and jumpy, his heart rate may increase, he may tremble and he may sweat. In extreme cases (e.g. soldiers before battle) he may lose control of urination or defaecation.

c. **Verbal expression.** He can describe his state of mind; he can tell others he is afraid.

Dogs can never provide verbal evidence of their fear, but they can provide the other two kinds of evidence; it is, therefore, in no way anthropomorphic to attribute fear to a dog. It is reasonable to assume that a dog is afraid of a particular situation if:

a.   it tries to escape from the situation or deliberately avoids it or

b.   it shows signs of high arousal, i.e. trembling, panting, whining or urinating involuntarily.

Some fear reactions are instinctive; most animal species react instinctively with a degree of fear to something completely novel or to a mixture of the familiar and the unexpected. Thus a puppy may show fear of its owner if, for example, she puts on a hat for the first time. In addition, some dogs of the same breed share a tendency to react with fear to the same specific stimulus. For example, in Border collies it is fairly common to find a fear of men waving sticks. This breed specificity implies an inherited instinctive component to the fear. **Most fear reactions are learned,** however. According to learning theory, they are acquired by the mechanism of classical conditioning (Chapter 3.1). Responses of the autonomic nervous system (unconditioned response) which are originally evoked by an unpleasant or startling stimulus (unconditioned stimulus) can later be elicited as a conditioned response to stimuli which were present at the same time as the painful stimulus. The classic demonstration of a fear response acquired in this way by a human being was by Watson (1920), one of the early behaviourists. He gave an 11-month-old boy, Albert, a white rat to play with, having previously made sure that the boy was not afraid of it. Then, whenever the boy reached for the rat, the experimenter made a loud startling noise behind him. After about five repetitions of this procedure, the boy began to show fear of the rat. Subsequently the fear generalised to similar furry objects, such as white rabbits and cotton wool. A similar process has frequently been experimentally demonstrated in animals. For example, Wolpe (1952) induced a phobic reaction in cats by putting them in experimental cages and administering electric shocks; subsequently, the more similar was the cage they were put in to the experimental cage, the greater was the intensity of their fear.

Dogs can acquire fears in the normal course of events by a similar mechanism. If a dog undergoes a painful or unpleasant procedure at the hands of a veterinary surgeon, the autonomic responses evoked may subsequently be evoked merely by the sight of the veterinary surgeon or his consulting room. This fear may also generalise to other veterinary practitioners and their premises: i.e. to other people in white coats and to other places with a similar smell.

5.2. GENESIS OF PHOBIAS

Most of the fears learned in this way are unlearned in the normal course of events. As Albert met more and more furry things which were not accompanied by unpleasant experiences, his fear probably diminished. Similarly, most dogs which develop a fear of their veterinary surgeon will cease to be so afraid after a few pleasant and reassuring encounters with him; this is the normal process of extinction as described in Chapter 3.9. However, **in a few cases fears do not extinguish;** the fear remains at the same high level for months or years, even though the conditioned stimulus is never paired again with the noxious unconditioned stimulus. These fears are known as phobias. Common examples of phobias among people are fear of being in enclosed spaces or fear of insects. Common examples of phobias in dogs are fear of the sound of gunfire, fear of traffic or fear of a particular kind of person, for example men.

The important question about phobias is why the fear persists in this way.**There are several possible reasons.**

a.   **The original unconditioned stimulus was of traumatic proportions.** In a study by Solomon & Wynne (1953), dogs were placed in a special cage in which they first of all heard a buzzer and then received an electric shock which they could escape by jumping a barrier. The difference between this unpleasant experiment and others concerned with the effect of punishment was that the shock was a very painful one. After this experience, the dogs always jumped over the barrier when they heard the buzzer, even though the buzzer was never again paired with shock, over hundreds of trials.

Similar reactions can be seen in people who have undergone horrific experiences. For example, the policeman who was a hostage in the Iranian embassy, interviewed several months afterwards, reported that he still felt sick with anxiety if he encountered the smell of the after-shave lotion used by one of the terrorists.

It is common for owners of phobic dogs to attribute the genesis of the phobia to a single traumatic incident and, as we have just seen, this is theoretically possible. However, in the author's experience, few of these traumas have actually been witnessed; most of them are reconstructions after the event. For example, the owner of a 5-year-old Labrador retriever with a phobia of the sound of gunfire, reported that the phobia had suddenly started when there had been a lot of shooting of game near her house. She presumed that the dog had been shot at but had no direct evidence of this. Although, like most of the reconstructions, it is a plausible explanation, the fact that so few of these incidents have been witnessed may imply that they occur less often than is supposed.

b. **In many cases, the experience of fear itself is so unpleasant that it operates as an unconditioned stimulus.** For example, frightened air travellers may not need an external event, such as a near-disaster, to maintain their fear: the internal events of churning stomach, pounding heart and mental images of disintegrating aircraft, are enough. This phenomenon might be called 'being afraid of fear'. It seems reasonable to suppose that a similar mechanism (without the mental images) operates in the case of canine phobias.

5.3. TREATMENT OF PHOBIC ANXIETY

Many owners unsuccessfully try to treat their dogs' fears by forcing them into the feared situation, with the aim of 'showing him it's alright'. For instance, the owners of a bearded collie with a fear of going out of the house, especially for walks, had tried to treat the problem by physically dragging it out of doors every day. This manoeuvre rarely works. Ordinary fears are usually unlearned in the normal course of events without the owner having to do anything about it. If an owner feels compelled to try to treat the problem, it usually means that the fear has reached the proportion of a phobia and cannot, for one or more of the reasons given above, be unlearned simply by repeated presentations of the conditioned stimulus without the unconditioned stimulus. Also, the experience of being forced against one's will into a situation probably adds to the unpleasantness of the whole experience. Thus, every time the owner in the above example took the bearded collie outside, the conditioned stimulus (being outside) was probably paired with two kinds of unpleasant unconditioned stimulus (a) the autonomic sensations of extreme anxiety and (b) the feeling of being dragged along against its will.

It should be mentioned that a method of treating phobias known as 'flooding' is sometimes used with human patients, whereby the patient is forced to remain in the feared situation until the physiological fear responses are exhausted. There are, however, two drawbacks to this method. First, it is extremely unpleasant for the patient. Secondly, it can sometimes back-fire and the patient can end up more fearful than he was originally.

The behavioural method most commonly used for the treatment of human phobias is '**systematic desensititization**'. It involves teaching or inducing the patient to perform some response which is incompatible with anxiety, in the presence of the feared stimulus. In theory, a whole range of behaviour could be employed as the incompatible response, such as sexual behaviour or eating but, in practice, relaxation is the response most often used. The patient is first taught, over several sessions, to relax, until eventually he can achieve a state of deep relaxation. A graded list or hierarchy of phobic stimuli is then drawn up, starting with stimuli which make the patient only slightly anxious and ending with those which make him panic-stricken. Thus, for a patient with a phobia of wasps, the hierarchy might start with the sight of a single wasp at a distance and end with a dozen angry wasps buzzing round her head. The weakest stimulus in the hierarchy is then presented to the patient while she is in a state of relaxation. Because of obvious practical difficulties, imagining the stimulus is often used as a substitute for the real thing; perhaps surprisingly, the generalisation to the real life situation is usually very good. Because she is relaxed, the patient can normally tolerate the milder phobic stimuli with little anxiety. As the treatment proceeds, stronger and stronger stimuli are presented and, if it proceeds slowly and gradually enough, they too will evoke little anxiety, until eventually even the strongest item in the hierarchy can be tolerated without undue anxiety. A similar method can be used to treat phobias in dogs. The responses incompatible with anxiety which are most often used are relaxation (induced by petting and soothing words from the owner), eating (feeding the dog tit-bits in the presence of the feared object) or playing with a favourite toy. For a fuller explanation of this technique see Chapter 8.

5.4. STATES OF HIGH AROUSAL

Because of avoidance or attempts to escape, it is fairly easy to tell when a dog or person has a fear of a specific stimulus. A person or a dog can also get into states of high arousal, the autonomic components of which are similar to fear, but which do not involve an avoidance reaction to a specific stimulus. People may describe the subjective experience of being in such a state as 'on edge', 'psyched up', 'excited' or 'anxious'. Although the state may be experienced as subjectively pleasant or unpleasant according to the situation, the psysiological accompaniments of all these states are similar: restlessness, alertness, increased heart-rate and increased gastro-intestinal motility.

MANIFESTATIONS OF HIGH AROUSAL

The same states of generalised high arousal can also be seen in dogs and are described by their owners as 'excited', 'going crazy', or 'highly strung' etc. They may be manifested behaviourally in some of the following ways:

a. **Alertness:** the dog responds excessively to external stimuli. A slight noise in another room, for instance, may send it dashing to investigate.

b. **Restlessness:** the dog may dash from room to room or run round in circles.

c. **Vocalisation:** the dog may bark or whine.

d. **Urination and defaecation:** the dog may urinate or defaecate very frequently out of doors. It may even urinate or defaecate indoors if it cannot get out or if the excitement is extreme.

e. **Increase in attachment.** When frightened or anxious, people generally want to be with their nearest and dearest. In the same way, an anxious dog may follow its owner from room to room or be more sensitive to cues that the owner is about to leave the house.

f. **Displacement activities:** this is an ethological term to describe parts of an instinctive behaviour pattern which are performed out of context and which seem to have a tension-relieving function for the animal. They are typically performed when the animal's state of high arousal is due to a conflict between two drives (see 5.8) or to frustration in the performance of some instinctive activity (as when an adversary suddenly flees in the middle of a fight). Common displacement activities in dogs are scratching, grooming, sexual mounting of inanimate objects, tail-chasing, chewing and digging. To be classed as such, the activity must be performed in isolation, not as part of a sequence which makes sense. So a dog which carries a bone away into a corner and chews it is not engaged in a displacement activity, but a dog which suddenly chews its foot may be. A displacement activity which is performed in a repetitive way is often referred to as a 'stereotypy'.

Displacement behaviour may pose problems for the owner. It is necessary to be aware that it may be a manifestation of high arousal, as in that case its treatment must include some reduction of the underlying anxiety or excitement.

These states of high arousal can be caused by various factors, usually operating in combination.

5.5 CAUSES OF HIGH AROUSAL

a. **Instinctive response to specific stimuli.** The fact that some kinds of stimuli so commonly and meaninglessly evoke an excited response suggests that some dogs have an inherited propensity to respond to these stimuli. For example, a high pitched noise, such as the telephone ringing, commonly provokes excitement.

   Dogs also possess, in varying degrees, the tendency to respond instinctively with anxiety to more complex situations which imply insecurity. Thus, a puppy may become upset if put in a strange environment and an adult dog may become anxious if separated from its owner.

b. **Learned response to specific stimuli.** Stimuli which are habitually associated with a state of excitement can quickly come to evoke excitement on their own. Some dogs start barking and dashing up and down when their owners fetch their leads, or when their food bowls are produced. Similarly, some dogs become uncontrollably excited in the car because they associate it with an imminent walk. The excitement in these cases is probably increased because there is an element of frustration; the stimuli of lead or food bowl signals gratification, but at that point the gratification is still delayed.

   In most cases where a dog becomes acutely agitated or excited some precipitating stimulus, either learned or instinctive, is present. When the excitement is episodic, the stimulus is usually fairly easy to identify: a loud noise, for example, or visitors coming to the house. Where the excitement is a more constant feature of the dog's behaviour, the stimulus may be less easy to identify; one possibility always worth investigating is that the stimulus is the owner's presence.

CASE EXAMPLE 5.1:

A three-year-old Staffordshire Bull Terrier was brought for treatment by a man in his forties. The problem was that for the last six weeks, ever since the dog had been castrated, it had spent most of its waking hours chasing its tail. It whirled round and round in a frenzied way, banging into things and, to all appearances, oblivious of what was going on around it. The owner was extremely upset and angry. He would only talk of his conviction that the referring veterinary surgeon had bungled the operation in some way and that the dog was still in pain. In an attempt to identify some triggering stimulus for this behaviour, the dog was taken away from its owner into another room. The intensity of the whirling diminished markedly and it eventually stopped. When the dog was brought back to its owner, the whirling immediately started again.

Although episodes of excitement are usually precipitated by a particular stimulus, they are also made more likely by various other factors which can increase a dog's general level of arousal (see 5.7c, d, e and f).

c. **A state of high drive.** According to learning theory, we are all motivated by drives of various kinds. Some of these are drives based on bodily needs and urges, such as hunger, thirst, sex and so on. By and large these drives based on physical needs grow stronger the longer they remain unsatisfied. The stronger the drive motivating an animal, the more aroused it becomes and the more likely it is to be excited by stimuli unconnected with the drive. For example, quite a high proportion of pet dogs are kept short of exercise. In a breed which needs exercise, the longer the dog goes without it, the more likely it will be to get anxious and agitated. It may bark at slight sounds or become destructive if its owner goes out.

d. **Conflict.** Animal experiments have shown that if an animal is under the influence of two conflicting drives, this itself increases anxiety. The greatest anxiety is produced when the animal is both attracted to and repelled from the same object: an approach/avoidance conflict. Thus, if a rat is taught to run a maze, is rewarded with food at the end of it and is then given an electric shock as it is eating the food, it will develop a conflict about going to the end of the maze; it will stop at some distance from the goal box, showing signs of anxiety and even, in the case of some rats, having fits.

In dogs, one of the most commonly seen approach/avoidance conflicts is one with the owner as focus. A dog's attachment to its owner is usually imprinted by contact with him as a puppy. It is difficult subsequently to break that attachment. If an owner is nasty to his dog, the dog usually develops conflicting feelings about the owner, with a consequent rise in anxiety. A circumscribed form of that conflict can be seen in 'hand-shy' dogs, which, when called, approach the owner but stop some distance away. The dog may show its state of conflict by barking or looking agitated.

Another kind of conflict which can produce great anxiety is a situation in which the subject has to make a difficult decision in order to avoid an unpleasant stimulus. Shengar-Krestovnikova (1921) demonstrated this phenomenon in dogs. Using food as the unconditioned stimulus, she conditioned a salivary reflex to the presentation of a picture in a circle; using electric shock to the forepaw, she conditioned paw withdrawal to a picture of an elipse. She then made the elipse and circle more and more similar in shape, so that in order to 'predict' what would happen next the dogs had to make more and more difficult discriminations. When the discrimination became too difficult, the dogs 'broke down', yelping, trembling and trying to escape.

Some pet dogs encounter similar situations when they are treated inconsistently by different members of the same family or by the same owner on different occasions. Thus, some family members may welcome the dog beside them on the sofa, whereas others may shout at it if they find it there. In the same way an owner may be pleased to be jumped on exuberantly by the dog when he feels relaxed and sociable, but if he is preoccupied he may become cross with the dog for doing the same thing. Most dogs experience a certain amount of this inconsistency from their owners; they often learn by subtle cues to distinguish the occasions when a certain behaviour will be approved of and when it will not. If there is conflict and upheaval within the family or if an owner is himself neurotically disturbed (see Chapter 7.4), the inconsistency may reach such proportions that the unpredictability of its life makes it extremely anxious.

e. **Confinement.** It has also been shown that confining an animal increases the effect of an anxiety-producing situation. Thus, an animal given an electric shock or called on to make a difficult discrimination will appear more anxious or will 'break down' much more quickly if it is restrained in a harness. This is presumably because the restless behaviour and displacement activities which an unconfined and anxious animal displays have the function of reducing its anxiety somewhat.

Confinement may be a factor contributing to the excitement which some dogs show in cars, from which there is no escape. It also may be a factor contributing to the destructiveness which some dogs display when left alone. In many cases the destructiveness is a displacement activity prompted by anxiety at being separated from the owner (see Chapter 10.6). Often the anxiety and, therefore, the destructiveness seems to be increased by confining the dog. Some owners, for example, who had previously given the dog the run of the house and had returned to find valuable furniture damaged, try to solve the problem by shutting the dog in the kitchen or bathroom. This may exacerbate the problem and increase destructiveness. Owners who try to solve the problem by giving the dog more freedom, for example access to the garden, often meet with more success. As confinement is usually ony a contributory factor in these cases, the dog's anxiety cannot usually be entirely eliminated by giving it more freedom. This method of treatment, therefore, should be used with discretion and only as an adjunct to the main treatment which should be aimed at reducing the dog's separation anxiety.

f. **Personality.** It is clear that **some dogs are temperamentally more disposed than others to develop phobias or behaviour disorders of excessive excitement** such as barking in cars. Some of the owners of dogs suffering from these disorders report either, in the case of phobias, that the dog has always been nervous, withdrawn and inclined to shy away from things or, in the case of excitement, that it has always been 'highly strung', jumpy or hyperactive.

This variation in what can be termed emotionality or neuroticism is found in many animals, including man. There is good evidence that it is mediated by differences in the reactivity of the autonomic nervous system (Eysenck, 1960). There is also evidence that there is an inherited factor in such differences. For example, Shields, (1962) found a significant correlation on a questionnaire test of neuroticism between pairs of monozygotic twins brought up separately. In the case of dogs, Murphree, *et al*, (1967) developed, by selective breeding over a single generation, two strains of pointers, one stable and the other neurotic whose behaviour differed significantly on experimental tests.

The role of early experience in causing predisposition to later neurosis is still a matter of controversy where human being are concerned. In the case of dogs, the evidence is clearer; puppies reared in a socially or environmentally impoverished environment are more likely to grow into neurotic dogs (see Chapter 6.2).

There remains the question why some neurotic dogs react with fear and others with excitement to the same stimuli. It seems likely that, as in man, this variation is due to differences on another personality dimension: introversion/extraversion. It is well established that when human subjects answer personality questionnaires, factor analysis of the responses usually yields two factors. The first is neuroticism, which has already been referred to, and the second is introversion/extraversion. Extraverts are typically sociable, impulsive people and introverts tend to be more thoughtful and withdrawn. These personality differences can also be demonstrated in subjects' performance on certain laboratory tests. For example, introverts tend to make fewer mistakes and are able to concentrate for longer.

This dimension of introversion/extraversion can also be applied to dogs. Pavlov (1927) described a similar dimension, using the terms 'inhibition' and 'excitation'. Cattell (1973), factor analysing dogs' performance on laboratory tests, found a similar factor.

Using human subjects, Eysenck, (1964) showed that neurotic extraverts tend to manifest their neurosis in behavioural symptoms such as anti-social or self-destructive actions, whereas neurotic introverts tend to suffer from phobias or obsessional symptoms.

It seems likely, therefore, that dogs with neurotic disorders might be classified in the same way; that on the appropriate tests dogs with phobias, or those which are excessively shy or fearful, would perform as neurotic introverts, whereas those which are excitable or hyperactive would perform as neurotic extraverts. As yet the crucial experimental study has not been carried out, but, in the meantime, the conceptual framework which this hypothesis provides seems the most useful one now available for making sense of neurotic disorders in dogs (see Chapter 10).

The most important points of practical relevance implied by the theoretical discussion in this chapter are these:

1. **Most behaviour disorders in which anxiety plays a major causative role are partly a result of learned or instinctive reactions to specific stimuli.** By modifying the stimuli, or taking appropriate steps to bring about relearning something can often be done to modify the disorder.

2. These behaviour disorders are also often partly caused by a neurotic predisposing personality. Early environment may play a part in forming this personality. Genetic factors also play a part. This has two implications:

    a. **Owners of neurotic dogs should not hope to change their dogs' personality, merely to alleviate its more troublesome manifestations.** Also, where appropriate, it should be made clear to the owner that although he may have unwittingly contributed to the development or maintenance of a specific symptom, he is unlikely to be responsible for the dog's neurotic personality.

    b. **Breeders have a responsibility not to breed from anxious or excitable dogs (see also Chapter 12.1) and to provide an optimum environment for the puppies from a psychological point of view.**

FURTHER READING

SAUTER, F. J. and GLOVER, J. A. (1978). Behaviour, Development and Training of the Dog. Chapters 4 and 7. Arco Publishing Company, New York.

DEVELOPMENTAL PSYCHOLOGY

Chapter Six _____

First three weeks; socialisation period; development after fourteen weeks.

In comparison with other aspects of dog behaviour, a great deal is known about its development and about the effect of early experiences on later behaviour. Unfortunately, for the most part, this information is not applied where it would be most useful. Owners continue to buy puppies from pet-shops and puppy farms and many breeders continue to rear their puppies in kennels. It might be argued that the veterinary profession is the one best placed to publicise the relevant information and bring pressure to bear on breeders to apply it.

6.1. FIRST THREE WEEKS

For the first three weeks of life, the puppy's needs are basic and physical: food, warmth, rest and the reflex stimulation of urination and defaecation. It has a simple repertoire of reflex behaviour (e.g. the rooting reflex and negative geotaxic response) to enable it to satisfy those needs. The bitch also has a repertoire of instinctive behaviour (e.g. licking, lying down on her side, responding to puppies' cries) which dovetails with the puppies' repertoire.

One of a breeder's chief priorities, therefore, must be to maintain this bitch/puppy group as a functioning unit.

Anything which disturbs the bitch or interferes with the smooth operation of her instinctive behaviour may have a detrimental effect on the puppies.

During the first stage of labour a bitch often indicates the kind of place she considers most suitable as a nest for her litter. More often than not, this is a location quite unsuitable from the owner's point of view, under the tool-shed, perhaps, or in the linen cupboard. Some of its characteristics, however, can be replicated in a more suitable environment specially constructed for the purpose. The bitch is usually happiest in a small, enclosed space which is warm, dark and secluded. An insulated box with a lid in a quiet room normally meets these requirements. Heat should be provided by a heating pad rather than an overhead lamp, which tends to overheat the bitch. As far as possible, she should be left undisturbed; the owner should resist the temptation to show off the puppies to visitors. Any displays of maternal aggression, such as growling at people or other animals entering the room, should as far as possible be respected.

Owners of pet bitches which are very attached to them may encounter the problem of the bitch not settling alone with the puppies, but constantly seeking the owner's company. In these circumstances, scenes in which the owner reprimands the bitch, orders her back to the puppies and shuts the door are not productive and may make the bitch even more unsettled. It is better to try to discover a different living arrangement which suits the bitch better, such as siting the puppies in the living room or the owner spending more time in the bitch's room.

There is evidence from laboratory rodents that neonatal protein deficiency is associated with increased emotionality in later life (Hart & Hart, 1985). The owner should, therefore, be ready to give supplementary feeds to puppies which are not gaining weight at the same rate as the others.

As puppies at this age are unable to see or hear and show an EEG characteristic of sleep, they are largely shielded from the psychological effects of their environment. It has been shown, however, (Fox, 1965) that some degree of olfactory learning takes place, which presumably helps in bonding mother and puppy. For example, the bitch, by licking the new born puppies and her nipples, may give the puppies an olfactory cue which helps them to find their first feed.

Another implication of early olfactory learning is that early handling by the owner facilitates the formation of the canine/human bond. In addition, it has been shown that puppies subjected to mild physical stress in early life (flashing lights, changes in temperature and posture) are better at problem solving, show dominance over their litter mates and are more attracted to people (Fox and Stelzner, 1966). These results are consistent with the general finding that handling is beneficial for the young of various species. Breeders should, therefore, be encouraged to handle their young puppies. Most conscientious breeders do this anyway, but some may need reassurance that it is all right to do so: there is a school of thought which recommends keeping handling to a minimum.

6.2. SOCIALISATION PERIOD

At two to three weeks of age, the situation changes dramatically. **From the time that they can hear and see, start to explore and interact with each other, until they are twelve to fourteen weeks old, the puppies' physical and social environment can profoundly affect their later personality.** This period, from three to twelve weeks, is known as the socialisation period. More particularly the following processes take place:

a. **Interaction with litter-mates**

    During this time, puppies play intensively, practising their instinctive repertoire of social responses. Much of this social play is concerned with expressing dominance and submission and with discovering ways of gaining dominance or avoiding submission. It is likely that their social experience with their litter-mates at this stage has the following permanent effects:

    i.   **If a puppy is deprived of interaction with its litter-mates, for example if it is removed from its litter at six weeks or earlier, its behaviour towards other dogs may be disordered in later life.** It may be excessively fearful of other dogs or, more inconveniently, inappropriately aggressive (Chapter 9.8).

    ii. If a puppy is much larger or smaller than the rest of its litter-mates, it may consistently find itself in the dominant or in the subordinate position. It is likely that this experience affects a dog's tendency to assume a dominant or subordinate role towards other dogs or people in later life.

b. **Interaction with mother**

    Although she spends less and less time with her litter over the socialisation period, **it is likely that both the quality and duration of the bitch's interaction with her puppies has an effect on later behaviour.** Scott & Fuller, (1965) have shown that on various tests of emotionality, puppies tend to obtain scores more similar to their mothers' than their fathers'; it may, therefore, be inferred that nervous bitches tend to pass their nervousness on to their puppies behaviourally as well as genetically. In general, mammals which have been prematurely separated from their mothers when young are less socially competent as adults. There is more specific evidence that this is true of dogs (Fält and Wilsson, 1979).

c.   **Interaction with people**

A puppy has to be absolutely deprived of human contact up to the age of 14 weeks in order to make it as fearful in the presence of human beings as a wild animal. Scott & Fuller (1965) found that puppies reared in a home environment were more confident generally with human beings than were puppies reared in kennels with consistent but restricted human contact. Dogs which are fearful of people, or certain kinds of people, may turn out to have spent at least the early part of their socialisation period in a kennel or outhouse, only visited at intervals by human beings for physical care (see Case Example 7:5). It therefore seems advisable that **puppies from three weeks onwards should as far as possible be part of a human household,** interacting with a range of people including men, women and children.

d.   **Interaction with the environment**

It has been shown that puppies reared in extremely impoverished environments can show a wide range of impairments (Agrawal, *et al.,* 1967; Melzack & Scott, 1957) including impaired learning ability, hyperactivity and fearfulness. Thus, dogs which show fear of such things as vacuum cleaners or cars may turn out to have had limited experience of such phenomena during the socialisation period. **It therefore seems advisable as far as possible to expose a young puppy to a wide variety of everyday sights and sounds.**

Scott & Fuller (1965) showed that a puppy's tendency to approach new people and things is strongest at about five weeks of age and declines thereafter. It shows little fear of new people or things at this age, but this fear increases thereafter. If possible, therefore, **a puppy should be introduced to new experiences early in the socialisation period.**

It used to be thought that the 'critical' period for learning which occurs in the young of most species was strictly time-limited. It is now known that this differential capacity for learning is not all or nothing e.g. if puppies do not have adequate experience of human beings or other dogs in the first 3 months of life, this experience can be made up later, although normally much more exposure is needed at these later times.

It also seems that under certain conditions, such as stress, this learning can happen quickly, even in adult life: thus Bateson (1983) records the example of a Soay sheep, previously unsocialised to human beings, which underwent a difficult labour and subsequent Caesarian section; it thereafter followed people around. This stress-induced attachment is thought to be mediated by nor-adrenalin which facilitates neural plasticity. This suggests interesting possibilities in the treatment of dogs which have had inadequate socialisation experiences as puppies. Advantage could be taken of naturally occurring stress such as illness or surgery: during recovery the dog should be exposed to the relevant species.

There is also evidence (Bateson, 1987) that the part of the system which mediates learning of social attachments has a limited capacity and that different kinds of potential objects of attachment are in competition with one another; according to this model, biologically appropriate stimuli have preferential access to this system. The implication for the rearing of puppies is that too much exposure to other dogs may militate against attachment to people: it adds further emphasis to the recommendation that puppies should be given as much exposure as possible to people as early as possible. In addition, special care should be taken by owners when introducing puppy into a household with other dogs: if the owner does not interact sufficiently with the puppy, there is a danger that it will become preferentially attached to other dogs.

6.3: DEVELOPMENT AFTER 14 WEEKS

After the first three months, the puppy's personality continues to mature in a similar way, but at a slower rate. It becomes gradually less randomly active, less excitable and less indiscriminately friendly; it becomes gradually more cautious and able to inhibit or postpone intended actions.

Increased dominance

At the time of puberty, sexually related behaviour appears. Male dogs may make a bid for dominance at this time. At around two years of age, further personality changes are often seen. These are usually connected with increased dominance and are presumably related to hormonal changes; two years is the age at which wolves first become capable of breeding. Owners of male dogs of breeds inclined to dominance should be made aware of this phenomenon and encouraged to maintain strict dominance over their dogs at around this time.

Early training

Owners are frequently confused as to when they should start to 'train' their dogs, having perhaps been advised on the one hand that a dog cannot be trained until it is at least six months old and on the other that training cannot start too soon. The answer to this question depends on the response to be trained. From early in the socialisation period, puppies are capable of acquiring both classically conditioned and instrumentally learned responses (Chapter 3), provided that the responses are not too complex and provided that they involve learning to do something positive or getting accustomed to something rather than exercising self-control. Thus, young puppies can be taught to sit on command, but it is difficult for them to stay sitting. They can also be accustomed to walking on a lead and trained to come when called. Most importantly, the foundations of **house-training** start at three weeks, when puppies instinctively leave the nest to urinate or defaecate; puppies which are prevented from doing this may be more difficult to house-train later. At around eight weeks, the puppy will start to use predictable locations for urination and defaecation, sniffing the ground for scent marks before it relieves itself. It is at this time that house-training can begin in earnest. The owner should ensure that scent marks are left in an appropriate place by taking the puppy there at the times when it is likely to urinate or defaecate; after sleep, after food, every hour or so when it is awake and when the owner sees it sniffing for scent marks (see also Chapter 12.10).

FURTHER READING
SAUTER, F. J. and GLOVER, J. A. (1978). Behaviour, Development and Training of the Dog. Chapter 3. Arco Publishing Company, New York.
SCOTT, J. P. and FULLER, J. L. (1965). Genetics and the Social Behaviour of the Dog. University of Chigago Press.

OWNER ATTITUDES

Chapter Seven _____

**Factor analytic studies;
psychological functions of owner-dog relationships;
owner personality and perception of dog behaviour;
effect of owner's personality on dog behaviour;
modifying owner's attitudes.**

Veterinary practitioners are constantly being made aware that owners' attitudes towards their dogs vary enormously. Some owners are so attached to their dogs that they are willing to travel the length of the country and spare no expense to obtain the appropriate specialist treatment for them, while others frustrate the veterinary surgeon's efforts by their unwillingness to pay even for routine procedures and by their negligence in carrying out instructions.

It should be evident from the previous chapters that a dog's behaviour is influenced in many ways by that of its owner. As an owner's behaviour towards his dog is obviously to some extent determined by his attitude towards it and the nature of his relationship with it, it is necessary to take these aspects of human psychology into account when studying canine behaviour.

7.1. FACTOR ANALYTIC STUDIES OF OWNER ATTITUDES

Wilbur (1976) gave a questionnaire to 350 dog owners in the USA, asking them about their attitudes towards their dogs. He found that the responses indicated five categories of owner. There were 'companion' owners (27% of the total) who regarded their dogs as members of the family; 'enthusiastic' owners (17%) who enjoyed their dogs but showed a less close involvement with them; 'worried' owners (24%) who were attached to their dogs but were worried or embarassed by their behaviour; 'valued object' owners (19%) who seemed to have no emotional tie with their dogs but viewed them as possessions; 'dissatisfied owners' (19%) who derived no satisfaction from their dogs and found them to be purely a nuisance. These results indicate that one of the main dimensions along which attitudes vary is **degree of attachment** to the dog, the 'companion' owners being extremely attached, the 'dissatisfied' owners not at all. The results also indicate that there is another independent dimension: **degree of enjoyment** of the dog. The 'companion' owners are both attached and enjoy their dogs, while the 'worried' owners are in the unfortunate position of being attached to but not enjoying their dogs. Almost all owners of dogs showing behaviour problems which are seen by specialists are in this latter category, as they would not go to the trouble and expense of a specialist referral if they were not attached to their dogs. Veterinary surgeons also have to deal with the 'dissatisfied' owners who, because their degree of attachment to their dogs is low, are often interested in a 'magic' cure which involves neither trouble or expense. The veterinary surgeon often cannot interest these clients in behavioural treatment: he may be placed in the distressing position of having to destroy a dog when he could offer treatment which might have saved it.

7.2. PSYCHOLOGICAL FUNCTION OF OWNER-DOG RELATIONSHIPS

Although studies of the kind just described, which involve giving standardised questionnaires to groups of people, can yield informative results, there are certain aspects of owner attitudes to which they can never do justice. For example, a group study cannot reflect the complexity of each individual's relationship with his dog.

Many owners show inconsistent behaviour or attitudes towards their dogs. For example, some act and speak at times as if they were extremely attached to their dogs and at other times they neglect them or abuse them.

CASE EXAMPLE 7:1.

Danger, a two-year-old Labrador retriever cross was brought for treatment by Mrs. D. who reported he had attacked her husband. Mrs. D. was confined to a wheel chair, but had travelled from another city at considerable inconvenience and expense. Although the dog had various unpleasant and inconvenient habits besides his aggression (e.g. he regularly helped himself to meat from the freezer, which he had learned to open) she said she was extremely attached to him and would not consider parting from him, even though she recognised her marriage relationship was suffering. It was subsequently learned from the referring veterinary surgeon that this client was well known in the neighbourhood and had frequently been seen, together with her husband, systematically hitting and kicking the dog until he howled. There is no position on two dimensions of degree of attachment and tough-minded vs tender-minded attachment which would adequately define that woman's relationship with her dog.

Owners may also show grief reactions which they recognise are inappropriate.

CASE EXAMPLE 7:2

Mrs. E. consulted me because she had become depressed following the death, from heart failure, of her three year old cavalier King Charles spaniel bitch, Emma. Since the dog's death, she had suffered from insomnia, loss of appetite and a general feeling of hopelessness. She thought about Emma constantly and wept often. She told me she had lost her sister two years previously. They had been very close. Although she had been sad and had mourned her sister, she had not felt as if the world had come to an end, as she did now. She knew there was something odd about her reactions and this added to her distress: she feared that she might be going mad.

In addition, factor analytic studies of this kind cannot answer the question 'Why are people attached to their dogs; what is the psychological function of the attachment?' Many answers have been proposed. It is often suggested that a relationship with a dog is a substitute for a relationship with another human being. The role which owners are most often conscious of enacting is that of parent, with the dog as child. As Beck & Katcher (1983) have pointed out, however, the roles may also be reversed with the dog providing the owner with the unconditional affection and acceptance which a mother usually offers her child.

Beck & Katcher have also pointed out that owners often behave towards their dogs very much as young children behave towards a special cuddly toy such as a teddy bear. They use it for comfort when they need it, hugging, fondling and talking to it. On the other hand the dog may be ignored for long periods when this kind of comfort is not necessary, just as a child may leave a teddy-bear quite happily in the cupboard when he is busy playing. On occasions a child may take out his anger at something else by hitting his cuddly toy and throwing it across the room; most owners would admit that they sometimes shout at their dogs when it is really someone else in the family who has made them angry.

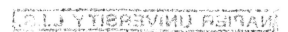

Serpell (1983), however, has argued that it may be dangerous to assume that a relationship with a pet is a substitute for another relationship. This would imply that the pet owner is psychologically less healthy than someone who engages in the 'real' relationship. Studies such as that by Hyde *et al*, (1983) have found little difference between the personalities of pet-owners and non-owners.

In applying all this to an individual owner in a clinical situation, it is necessary to bear in mind that people's relationships with their dogs vary so enormously that it seems likely that **the dog fulfils different psychological functions for different people.** For one thing, as factor analytic studies of owner attitudes have demonstrated, some people have so little psychological investment in their dog that its psychological function in their life must be minimal.

For those clients who are strongly attached to their dogs, and therefore to whom the dog is obviously psychologically important, the following formulation is often useful in conceptualising the part played by the dog in their mental life: **a dog is often felt to be not so much another person as an extension of the owner himself.** The dog is, therefore, seen as having the same personality characteristics as the owner; sometimes characteristics the owner is happy to possess and share with another, such as friendliness or playfulness; sometimes characteristics the owner is not comfortable with and may not even admit to himself that he possesses, such as aggressiveness or destructiveness. The nearest analogy is not a child and his teddy bear but a child and his imaginary companion. Children who have such companions at times talk of them as if they were mirror images of themselves, sharing all their activities and lending moral support to their likes and dislikes ('Bobby and I like getting wet'). At other times, the companion may be used to express controversial views ('Bobby says he likes white bread better than brown bread') or feelings of which the child feels ashamed ('Bobby doesn't like going to sleep in the dark').

Support of this view of attached owners' relationships with their dogs comes from owners' own statements, particularly when expressing grief after the death of a dog. They often say things like 'He was part of me' or 'I feel like I had lost an arm or a leg'. When talking about their dogs' likes and dislikes, it sometimes becomes clear that owners are attributing their own feelings to their dogs, rather than describing some behaviour they have observed in the dog, as with the owner who said of her Scottish terrier 'Gerald absolutely adores gardening and horses'. Also, when talking about a dog to which they are particularly attached, owners often feel that the communication between them is literally telepathic: one owner described how she could 'think' her dog upstairs in the morning.

In addition, **the projection into the dog of feelings which the owner finds difficult to cope with in himself is sometimes evident when the owner is finding the dog's behaviour problematic.**

CASE EXAMPLE 7:3.

A Mrs. F. brought a five-year-old spayed cairn Terrier bitch Fanny, complaining that the dog was prone to growl and snap when patted. This was particularly worrying to Mrs. F. as she ran a hotel and Fanny was often approached by guests. It also emerged that the dog had a habit of going under the desk in Mrs F's office; if she sat down to work, Fanny would growl until Mrs. F. was forced to withdraw. In addition, Fanny would not eat her meals if there was anyone in the kitchen with her; she would growl at them until they left.

It seemed that much of the problem was due to dominance aggression and various ways of reversing the dominance were discussed with Mrs. F. (see Chapter 9.2). She was encouraged to ignore the dog most of the time and reward with her attention only the obedient, submissive actions. She was also advised not to allow Fanny under the desk in the first place and to prevent her from guarding her food by hand-feeding her. She readily agreed to all this but, when she was seen again two weeks later, she reported no improvement. On further enquiry, she admitted that she had not made much effort to carry out the instructions; she said she felt Fanny had a right to be alone at meal times and to have some privacy under the desk. It also became evident from the way she talked about the dog,

51

speaking in an indulgent way about how naughty she had been, that although the behaviour was highly inconvenient, the owner partly relished it and did not condemn it altogether. When more was eventually learned about Mrs. F.'s domestic situation, the reason for this attitude became clearer. Two years before, her husband had had a stroke which disabled him, leaving her to look after the hotel and him single-handed. She also had a teenage son who did not help her much. In addition her general practitioner, she felt, had been particularly unhelpful about arranging rehabilitation and hospital admissions to give her a rest. It emerged that, altogether, she felt at everyone's beck and call and unable to demand help to which she was entitled. This made her feel very resentful about the whole situation. Her attitude towards Fanny was explained by the fact that she gave her some vicarious satisfaction by being able to do what she would have liked to do but could not. She would have liked to have had some peace and privacy to eat her meals, she would have liked to snap at the hotel guests sometimes and she would have liked to tell people to get out of the office when she was doing the accounts.

The idea that owners attribute their own feelings and personality characteristics, both desirable and undesirable, acknowledged and unacknowledged, to their dogs receives further support from the fact that this kind of attribution occurs between human beings. In the case of characteristics we like and are willing to admit, it has been shown by social psychologists that we tend to feel that our friends are similar in personality to ourselves. In the case of more problematic emotions, it is common in psychotherapeutic work with human patients to discover the kind of projection of unwanted emotions which was described earlier.

CASE EXAMPLE 7:4.

A woman in her twenties, married with a child of three, was referred to a psychologist because she was distressed by thoughts which kept coming into her head. These thoughts were that her husband was going to attack her or that he was being unfaithful to her. In fact, he was a quiet, passive man who had always behaved towards her in a dutiful, devoted way. On the other hand, he did not offer her much support in her emotional crises, being himself very anxious and prone to stomach pains. She had in the past formed a great attachment to a tutor at college who had given her the support her husband was unable to provide and she showed the same tendency to become extremely dependent on her general practitioner. In addition, she and her husband disagreed about having another child; she very much wanted another but he felt he could not cope with any more. She said she now accepted this and felt no bitterness towards him. It was evident that the intrusive thoughts which so distressed her were a result of having projected onto her husband both her wish to find another more satisfactory man (i.e. be unfaithful to him) and her anger with him for denying her another baby; thus, it now felt to her as if he were the violent and unfaithful one.

7.3. OWNER PERSONALITY AND PERCEPTION OF DOG BEHAVIOUR

To extend this theory of owner/dog relationships further, it would seem to follow that **an owner with a more stable personality is more likely to have the type of relationship in which he attributes to his dog characteristics, such as friendliness, which he acknowledges in himself, whereas an owner with personality problems is more likely to have the type of relationship in which he attributes to his dog the more problematic characteristics which he cannot acknowledge in himself.** Moreover, it also seems to follow that the former type of relationship is likely to be a satisfactory one, whereas the latter is likely to be more difficult, with the owner attributing to the dog behaviour problems, either real or imagined.

An experimental test of this view was carried out at the Royal (Dick) School of Veterinary Studies (O'Farrell, 1983). Twenty dog owners, attending the Small Animal Practice Teaching Unit for veterinary treatment, were asked to rate their own and their dog's personalities on 24 adjectives such as nervous, intelligent, aggressive: adjectives which could be applied to both dogs and human beings. The results showed a correlation between owners' ratings of themselves and of their dogs, indicating that, on the whole, owners see their dogs as being like themselves. Each owner was also asked to rate, on the same scales, 'Myself as I would like to be' i.e. his ideal self. It has been shown (Ryle & Breen, 1972) that the degree of discrepancy between ratings of self and ideal self correlates well with other measures of personality disturbance; neurotic patients, for example, tend to see themselves as less like they would wish to be than do normal subjects. The results showed that, as predicted, more stable subjects perceived their dogs as having more similar personalities to their own than did the subjects with more personality disturbance. The subjects who themselves showed more personality disturbance, also perceived their dogs as having more behaviour problems as rated on specific scales such as 'aggressive', 'nervous' or 'disobedient'.

This theory, that owners who are attached to their dogs tend to relate to them as if the dogs were an extension of themselves, can explain some phenomena which have to be recognised when studying relationships between dogs and people. Owners are often embarrassed to reveal the extent of their attachment to their dogs. A high proportion of owners, when alone, talk to their dogs in baby talk or as if they were human adults, but most feel embarrassed if they discover they are overheard. It could be argued that people feel rather embarrassed about their attachments to their dogs because somewhere inside themselves they realise, usually without being able to put it into words, that they are relating to the dog as part of themselves and therefore, in a sense, the relationship with the dog is a fantasy relationship. Others are eager to talk at length about their dogs and their doings. This can have the curious effect on the listener of being at the same time embarrassed and bored. The same effect can be produced by people telling their dreams in a social context and the reason for the effect is the same: it is very personal information communicated in a kind of code. It is delivered is such a way that, in a social situation, to refuse to take the code at face value and to comment on its personal content would seem rude or intrusive.

This element of projection or fantasy is an important feature of pet-owner relations. Workers involved in 'companion animal studies' often play it down, either because they feel it detracts from the seriousness of their work or because they are themselves caught up in the fantasy. But the element of projection does not detract from the benefit and satisfaction that many people derive from a dog's companionship or the intensity of the grief which can be experienced when the dog dies.

Although there is probably an element of projection in most pet-owner relations, it is arguably greatest in dog-owner relationships. There are several reasons for this:

a.   The dog shows a variety of instinctive behaviour patterns: something to suit a variety of human psychological needs.

b.   Typical breed differences in behaviour make it possible for an owner to pick a dog which is likely to fit in with his own particular projections.

c.   The behaviour of most dogs is changed by their owners' behaviour towards them, so that they are capable of adapting even more closely to the owners' projections.

d.   Dogs show instinctive behaviour which openly displays most of the primitive emotions which people may find problematic and are driven to express in covert ways: attachment and dependency, aggression, greed and sexuality.

Clinical relevance

What is the relevance of all this to the diagnosis and treatment of behaviour problems? First, if the owner has an ambivalent attitude towards his dog's behaviour (i.e. although the behaviour may be inconvenient in many ways, in other ways it may suit him psychologically) he may not carry out treatment instructions properly, especially those which involve changing his own behaviour towards the dog (see Case Example 7:3 above). In addition, the extent to which he is troubled by some aspect of the dog's behaviour, the extent to which he perceives it as a problem, may be affected by the emotions which he attributes to the dog. The following case provides an illustration of both these points.

CASE EXAMPLE 7:5.

Mrs. M. sought treatment for an 18 month old German shepherd dog, Max, which had always been restless and active but a few months before had started to behave more strangely. When he was indoors he would run to and fro whining, or run in circles biting his tail; he often scratched at the door to be let out, but when he was let out he behaved in a similar way in the garden, whirling round and round on the grass, digging up the flower beds in a frenzied way and so on. This went on for most of the day and Max was calm only when Mrs. M. relaxed in the evening watching television.

Although it was not clear what had caused this agitated behaviour, it seemed likely that it was being maintained, at least partly, by being rewarded with attention from Mrs. M. From her own account, whenever the dog started to get excited, she would talk to him to try and calm him down; also there was no evidence that Max behaved abnormally when he was alone. Mrs. M. was advised that she should take care not to reward Max when he started to behave excitably; that she should either ignore him or put him away in another room, only letting him back with them when he had calmed down. When Mrs. M. was seen again she reported no improvement. It became clear from what she said that she was unable to ignore Max; she was too upset by his behaviour. Nor could she put him out of the room because she felt he was so deeply unhappy that to isolate him would be very cruel. In the discussion which followed, it emerged that she had always felt close to Max. She had named him after a brother with whom she had always felt a close bond and who had gone to live abroad. They had both shared an unhappy childhood but had relieved the misery by being able to confide in and support one another. A few months before, her brother, who had been unhappily married, had committed suicide. Mrs. M. still felt shattered by this loss; she also felt guilty that she had not been of more help to her brother, knowing how miserable he was.

It then turned out that Max had started to behave in an agitated way during the upset which immediately followed the brother's suicide. It also became clear that Max embodied for Mrs. M. the misery which she felt she and her brother had shared; Mrs. M. read into his hyperactivity all the unhappiness she supposed her brother to have suffered and which she also felt. At times, therefore, the dog's behaviour made her feel very solicitous and she paid it a great deal of affectionate attention, thus reinforcing and rewarding the abnormal behaviour. At other times, when she was trying to forget the whole thing and pull herself out of her misery, she could not stand the sight of Max, which she felt as a kind of albatross, a constant reminder of her own and her brother's misery; in this mood she might shout at Max and hit him. The effect of this inconsistent behaviour was almost certainly to make him more anxious (see Chapter 5.5d).

The outcome of this case was unfortunate. Shortly after she had been seen for the second time, Mrs. M. took Max to the veterinary surgeon for euthanasia, to which he immediately agreed. It emerged afterwards that she had had a letter from the wife of her dead brother which had made her feel particularly despairing about his death. She had felt suicidal, but instead of carrying out that impulse, had had the dog destroyed. She said "I knew I would only wake up in hospital if I took some pills, but at least I could put him out of his misery".

This could be described as an extreme and pathological example of the processes being discussed, but they can also be seen in a more subtle form in less disturbed clients. In the questionnaire study of 50 dog owners described in more detail below (O'Farrell, 1992), the owners were asked to complete the Neuroticism scale of the Eysenck Personality Inventory. They were also asked questions about possible behaviour problems in their dog and for each undesirable kind of behaviour (e.g. urinating in the house, biting people) they were also asked how much of a problem it was to them. For some behaviour there was a significant correlation between its frequency and how problematic it was to the owner; the correlations were highest (.7) for roaming, fighting with other dogs and destructiveness in the owner's absence; for some behaviour such as excitement with visitors, there was no correlation at all. This means that although there is some dog behaviour which most people find inconvenient, in many instances whether the dog's behaviour is a problem depends partly on other factors. That, in some cases, one of those factors is the owner's personality is confirmed by the finding that for the dog's fear of things such as thunder-storms or vacuum cleaners there was a significant correlation between the owner's Neuroticism score and the extent to which he found the dog's fears a problem, but no correlation between the Neuroticism scores and the actual frequency with which the dog displayed the behaviour. That is, the owner's own anxiety seems to play a part in determining how troubled he is by his dog's fears.

7.4. EFFECT OF OWNER'S PERSONALITY ON DOG BEHAVIOUR

So far, all that has been discussed is the effect the owner's personality and attitudes have on his interpretation of, and his reaction to, his dog's behaviour. There is the further interesting possibility that an owner's personality might also have a direct effect on his dog's behaviour and might be a causative factor in the development of behaviour problems. Results from the questionnaire study (O'Farrell, 1992) referred to above suggest that this might be the case. As well as completing a neuroticism questionnaire, the owners were also asked about their attitudes towards their dogs. In addition the owners were asked in some detail about possible behaviour problems. In order to obtain quantifiable information which was as objective as possible, for each problem area, they were asked specific questions about the frequency of the behaviour: i.e. not 'Does your dog bite people?' but 'How often does your dog bite people?'

When the scores on these items were factor-analysed, two main factors emerged. The first was a factor of dominance aggression. That is, growling at people, biting people, growling when patted or disturbed all tended to be associated and, if a dog showed one of these behaviours, he was more likely than average to show the others. The second factor is most appropriately labelled 'displacement activities', the items which loaded highest being 'Sexual mounting of inanimate objects or human beings' and 'Destructiveness when left alone' (see Chapter 5.4).

Factor analysis of the attitude items revealed two main factors: one was labelled 'attachment' (items loading highly were "I miss the dog when parted from him" and "dog sleeps in the bedroom"); the other was labelled 'anthropomorphic emotional involvement' (items loading highly were "dog is fed specially prepared food" and "I like a dog to be loving and dependent"). For each subject, a score on each of the four factors was calculated by summing the scores on the relevant items, weighted by their factor loadings. It was found that the aggression score was positively correlated with the emotional involvement score: that is, owners who were involved with their dogs in an anthropomorphic way were more likely than average to have dogs which showed dominance aggression.

In addition, owner neurosis was correlated with the 'displacement activity' factor. In other words, dogs whose owners were more anxious than normal were more likely to show displacement activities. These correlations do not demonstrate any causal connection between the variables but it is possible to speculate as to what these causal connections might be.

In the case of dominance aggression, as described in Chapter 4.7, research with various species which have dominance hierarchies suggests that one of the most important characteristics of a dominant animal is that it takes the initiative in social interaction. An owner who is emotionally attached to his dog is more likely to behave as if it is a friend and an equal than as if it is a subordinate. Therefore he will be likely to respond to the dog's initiatives and requests; if it barks to go out he will open the door; if it brings a ball he will play with it and so on. If the dog is predisposed to dominance by virtue of genetic or hormonal factors, it is likely to interpret this acquiescent behaviour of the owner as confirmation of its dominant status.

With regard to the connection between displacement activities in dogs and neurosis in the owners, it was pointed out in Chapter 5.4 that these displacement activities typically occur when the animal is in a state of conflict. The owner's high anxiety level may predispose him to use the dog as an object on which he can vent emotions which he cannot manage internally. This will lead him to behave inconsistently towards the dog, perhaps unpredictably rewarding and punishing the same action or alternately being affectionate and indifferent. As was pointed out in Chapter 5.8, this requires the dog to make impossible discriminations and is likely to induce in it a state of conflict and anxiety analogous to that produced experimentally by Shengar-Krestovnikova (1921). The hyperactive German shepherd dog of Case Example 7:5 would be an extreme example of this process.

7.5. OWNER ATTITUDES AND DIAGNOSIS

The question now arises of the relevance of these findings and theories to the diagnosis and treatment of dog behaviour problems. The first point is that **it is as important to recognise when an owner's attitude is not affecting the dog's behaviour as when it is affecting it.** It is often very tempting for a veterinary surgeon to dismiss a dog's problem as being due to the 'neurosis' of the owner; this mental manoeuvre absolves him from the effort of puzzling further over the causes of the problem and of devising a treatment plan. Clients themselves often unwittingly encourage a false solution of this kind. Although some detach themselves from their dog's problem, regarding it as an illness or defect in the dog and expecting it to be put right without any involvement on their part, the majority of clients referred to specialists feel excessively responsible for their dog's behaviour. They have taken to heart the often quoted maxim that there are no bad dogs, only bad owners.

In the majority of cases, there is evidence that the dog's behaviour is influenced by other factors, for example genetic, hormonal, early environment, which are quite outside the owner's control. In addition, even where the dog's behaviour is due to faulty learning, either as a result of the environment he has been placed in, or as a result of the owner inadvertently rewarding the undesirable behaviour, in many cases this cannot be ascribed to the owner's particular attitude as it involves behaviour which is typical of most owners and is compatible with a whole range of attitudes towards the dog. It is rather that this particular dog requires its owners to behave towards it in a special way, in order for it to function acceptably. In these cases it is usually not necessary to try to alter the owner's attitude towards the dog.

CASE EXAMPLE 7:6.

Miss P, a retired physiotherapist, particularly requested a home consultation because she suffered from agoraphobia. The problem was her nine month old corgi puppy, Pearl, who had developed a fear of going out of the house. In Pearl's case, this even extended to the garden: she would go out to urinate and defaecate, but then dash back into the house, without lingering to play. She was reluctant to go for walks round the block on a lead and could not be allowed to run freely in parks because of her tendency to dash for home.

Miss P. attributed the phobia to two traumatic events. At four months Pearl fell off a low wall in the garden onto her head. Around the same time, she was accidentally shut in a room by herself during a window cleaner's visit. Miss P. found her afterwards trembling behind a sofa. She noticed that thereafter Pearl was particularly afraid of metallic noises which resembled the clanking of a window cleaner's ladder.

Miss P. told me that some of her friends had made a link between her own agoraphobia and Pearl's problem: they told her that her own fear of going out had made Pearl afraid. However, it seemed that, on the contrary, Miss P.'s phobia was helpful to Pearl, rather than the reverse: empathising with Pearl, she did not force her into phobic situations which would have increased her fear. In fact, she had already started to systematically desensitize the dog by playing games with her in the garden.

7.6. MODIFYING OWNER ATTITUDES

Having formed a hypothesis as to the effect the owner's attitude is having on the dog, how does this affect the treatment? For an owner whose attitude seems unconnected with the dog's problem, it is often helpful to make this clear, as in Case Example 7:6. Even when his attitude seems to be making some contribution, it is often useful to make clear the limited nature of this contribution, also stressing the importance of, for example, genetic or hormonal factors, because this often makes it easier for the owner to make such changes as are necessary to his attitude or behaviour. It is much easier to change one's behaviour towards a dog if one feels one is being required to behave in a special way towards a dog with special problems than if one feels one is being called on to change one's attitude towards dogs in general.

When attempting to modify an owner's attitudes, it is useful to bear some points in mind. An owner's attitude towards his dog is a personal and sensitive subject; comments directed at changing those attitudes therefore have to be very carefully considered. If an owner senses that the veterinary surgeon condemns his attitude, he will be inclined to feel defensive and perhaps guilty. If the owner senses that the person advising him understands his feelings, he will be more inclined to be frank about what goes on between him and his dog; he will also be more open to pressure to make such changes are are necessary.

People cannot change their feelings voluntarily or just because they are told to do so. It is no use saying to someone 'You're too fond of that dog' or 'Your own anxiety makes that dog nervous'. Attitudes can be changed, however, by more indirect means:

a. **Altering the cognitive component**

The opinions which lie behind the attitude may be changed by giving information which is incompatible with the presently held attitude. Sometimes, informing the owner about some aspects of canine psychology can change his attitude towards his dog. For example, it is fairly common for owners of dogs which are destructive in their absence to feel that the dog is being spiteful or defiant. If it is explained to them that a dog is incapable of understanding a connection between the owner's anger and destruction carried out 3 hours previously, that the dog's apparent guilt is really fear of the punishment he has learned to expect (Chapter 2.4) and that the destruction is a manifestation of anxiety at being left alone (Chapter 10.7), then the owners often feel less hostile towards their dogs and are able to behave less inconsistently towards them.

b. **Altering the behavioural component**

For example, if the owner of a dog showing dominance aggression is instructed to ignore the dog most of the time, only paying attention to it when it obeys a command from the owner, this may not only influence the dog's perception of the owner, increasing the owner's dominance in the dog's eyes; it may also change the owner's attitude towards the dog. As a result of behaving towards the dog in a more detached way, the owner may begin to feel more detached from the dog; he may begin to regard it less as another human being and more of a dog.

c. **Insight**

More rarely, an owner's attitude can be changed by helping him towards some insight into his attitudes and behaviour towards the dog. This is possible with only a few clients and must be done tactfully and carefully, as most clients neither want nor expect comments on their own psychological processes. When this kind of change takes place it is more often as a result of the client working towards a new perspective himself, as a result of being able to discuss the dog and his feelings about it in a relaxed and understanding atmosphere, than as a result of having unwelcome truths thrust upon him.

CASE EXAMPLE 7:7.

Miss S. a young woman in her twenties sought treatment for Sammy, a black cocker spaniel with many problems; he urinated in the hall, he threatened the family (the owner's mother and sister) when they tried to carry meals to the table, he barked and screamed when taken on a bus or at certain places on the tenement stairway. The dog responded well to behavioural treatment up to a point. The aggression and inappropriate urination improved but did not entirely disappear. Some of the difficulty here seemed to lie in Miss S.'s inability to persuade her mother to modify her behaviour towards the dog, or to come to the consultations. Miss S. herself kept asking for further advice and consultations although it seemed that all that was possible at a behavioural level had been done. The comment was eventually made that Miss S. must find it very annoying that her mother would not do as she was asked. Miss S. then revealed that she suspected that her mother was becoming senile, but her GP would not take this suggestion seriously. She foresaw that she might become trapped into looking after Mrs S for many years to come. Her sister refused to discuss the situation and was making plans to go abroad. She then talked of how fed up she was with her mother; she herself owned the flat they lived in and she had (she now felt unwisely) invited her mother to stay there when she was widowed. There now seemed little prospect of Mrs S leaving, although they argued continually about details of running the household. As she talked she became aware that Sammy was a particular bone of contention between them. He was definitely Miss S.'s dog; Mrs S did not like dogs and was not willing to put herself out for it. Miss S. said little more on this visit, but she telephoned a few weeks later to report that the dog's behaviour was much improved. She said that as a result of the previous consultation she had spoken to her mother about the necessity for her to find her own home and they had more openly discussed the problems they had in living together. She said she thought she and her mother had been using Sammy and his bad behaviour to score points off each other, but now that they no longer needed to do so to the same extent, he was feeling less confused.

FURTHER READING

BECK, A. and KATCHER, A. (1983). Between Pets and People. C.P. Putnam, New York.

PART TWO

TREATMENT OF SPECIFIC DISORDERS

PRINCIPLES OF DIAGNOSIS AND TREATMENT

Chapter Eight

**Nature of diagnosis; taking a history;
formulating an explanation; treatment methods; surgery;
drugs; behavioural treatment; modifying owner attitudes.**

8.1. NATURE OF DIAGNOSIS

The diagnosis of behaviour problems requires a different approach from the diagnosis of physical problems. The client who presents a dog with a behaviour problem is asking for help with a domestic situation in which the behaviour of one of the family members (the dog) is causing difficulties. The difficulties are more often experienced by the human members of the family; more rarely the sufferer is the dog itself (as in the case of phobias) or another animal (as in the case of intraspecies aggression). Although it may be possible to give the dog's behaviour a descriptive label (e.g. phobia, dominance aggression), this label does not amount to an adequate diagnosis, in that it does not describe a clinical entity nor does it, on its own, enable effective treatment to be prescribed. For that to be possible, it is necessary to make an assessment of all factors operating, which differ in each individual case. Thus, in a particular case of dominance aggression, before effectively treating the problem, it might also be necessary to know (a) that it showed aggression towards certain family members only, (b) that the aggression was only shown in certain situations, (c) that there was a learned component in the aggressive response in that a successful confrontation by the dog often led to a reward, (d) that the dog was also under some stress because one family member was punishing it severely and inconsistently and (e) that another family member was extremely attached to the dog. **Rather than being content with assigning a diagnostic label to a behavioural problem, therefore, it is necessary to try to formulate an explanation of the dog's actions and the particular factors causing them.** When the term 'diagnosis' is used in the following text it is used to refer to this type of formulation.

Sometimes the differential diagnosis of a physical versus a behavioural problem presents itself. Because of their training, veterinary surgeons more often mistakenly label a behavioural problem as a physical problem rather than vice versa. It may be useful to bear in mind that the diagnoses are not necessarily mutually exclusive. For example, a dog already showing dominance aggression may show aggression more readily because it is suffering from an ear infection. Also, the more chronic the physical disorder, the more likely it is to acquire behavioural components: a dog which defaecates in the house because of a gastro-intestinal disorder may out of habit continue to do so after the gastro-intestinal condition has resolved. Dermatological disorders which the dog aggravates by licking or chewing may also benefit from a combined physical and behavioural approach.

8.2. TAKING A HISTORY

Because of the particular nature of the diagnostic process in behaviour problems, more information must be elicited from the client than is the case for most physical problems. Another reason why this is necessary is that the client is usually the main source of information about the problem, other sources such as physical examination or laboratory tests normally having little to contribute. Therefore, when investigating a behaviour problem, it is usually advisable to set aside a longer time than a veterinary surgeon would normally spend on a consultation. Behaviour problems are rarely so urgent that action has to be taken immediately. It may often be better to arrange to see a client again when more time can be spent in discussion, rather than try to reach a hasty formulation, conscious that other clients are being kept waiting.

In a diagnostic interview, it is usually advisable to cover the following areas (not necessarily in this order):

a. **Description of the problem**

   i. **What exactly does the dog do?**

   The clinician should not be content with a general description which can be ambiguous; 'nervous', for example, can mean 'reacts with hyperactivity or vocalisation to many stimuli' or 'shows fear in many situations' or 'is liable to bite'. An exact account should be obtained in terms of the dog's bodily postures, movements and vocalisations.

   ii. **In what situations does the behaviour occur?**

   Information on this point will help to determine the dog's motivation. For example, if a dog urinates in the house only when shut in the kitchen at night or when the owner is out, this raises the possibility that the urination is caused by separation anxiety. This information can also be important when planning treatment, as it can give some idea of the stimuli which trigger the behaviour; if there is a learned component in the behaviour, these stimuli may have to be modified (see 8.7).

   iii. **What happens following the behaviour?**

   The dog's behaviour afterwards is often not as important as the owner thinks it is. He may relate how the dog wags its tail or licks him after it has bitten, or how it crawls into a corner after an episode of destruction. He may feel that these are signs that the dog is at least showing some awareness that it has done wrong. Dogs frequently behave in bizarre ways following problem behaviour, because they have learnt to expect punishment at this point or because they are in a state of conflict between the drive which prompted the behaviour (e.g. aggression) and fear of punishment. Many of the so-called signs of remorse are displacement activities (see Chapter 5.4). On the other hand, information about what the owner does after the problem behaviour occurs can often provide additional clues about factors maintaining it. For example, if an owner reports that he usually comforts the dog when it behaves in a fearful manner, it is possible that the fear behaviour is at least in part an instrumentally learned response rewarded by attention.

b. **History of the problem**

   i. **When did the problem behaviour first occur?**

   This may give a clue as to possible causative factors. If the dog has shown the behaviour since it was a puppy, it is likely to have been influenced by genetic factors or early experience. If it first occurred around the time of puberty or the onset of adulthood (around 2 years), during oestrus, after spaying or castration, it is likely to be under hormonal influence.

ii. **Under what circumstances did the behaviour first occur?**

This can give some clue as to causative factors. For example, if a dog's owner has had a month of illness spent entirely at home and, when he returns to work, the dog starts to be destructive in his absence, it is likely that the destructiveness is at least in part caused by separation anxiety. It must be borne in mind, however, that behaviour which has originally appeared for one reason may continue for a different reason; for example, an originally 'genuine' phobic response may continue because it is rewarded by attention.

iii. **What have the owners already done to treat the problem?**

The dog's response to previous treatments often gives important information about causal factors. For example, if punishment has made it markedly worse, some state of anxiety or high arousal is probably involved. Response to previous treatments may also give some information as to what treatment may succeed in the future, but the clinician should not be diverted from undertaking the obvious treatment of choice without first making careful enquiries about the failed treatment. Especially in the case of behavioural treatments which involve relearning, details of the timing of the reward or the order in which stimuli are presented can make a crucial difference. For example, owners of phobic dogs will often report that they have tried what sounds like desensitisation; they have, perhaps, taken the dog into progressively more fear-provoking situations, while talking soothingly to it. On closer enquiry, however, it often emerges that the owner has allowed the dog to become too anxious in these situations and has then rewarded it with soothing words, a procedure which would reinforce the dog's phobic behaviour rather than desensitizing it.

c. **General information**

i. **What is the rest of the dog's behaviour like? Are there any other problems?**

There are two reasons for finding this out. One is that owners often initially present only one out of many problems. This may be to protect the clinician from feeling overwhelmed by an impossible case or it may be that the owner selects the problem which he thinks may be curable. However, it is necessary to know about all the problems at the outset, as they are often interconnected and must be tackled in a certain order. For instance, an owner may complain that his dog threatens visitors who come to the house, but in the interview it may emerge that the dog is also behaving in a dominant way towards family members. There is no point in trying to treat the aggression towards visitors without first or concurrently treating the dominance towards the family.

It is also important to know about the dog's general behaviour, whether problematic or not, as this can help with determining the causation or planning the treatment of the problematic behaviour. For example, the fact that a dog accepts attention and affection only on its own terms can help to confirm a diagnosis of dominance aggression. The treatment of a dog which barks and leaps about in the car is a more difficult prospect if it is generally excitable and hyperactive, than if this is the only situation in which it shows such behaviour.

ii. **What is the dog's daily routine?**

This question can elicit useful information about owner attitudes. For example, sleeping arrangements are often significant; an owner who lets the dog sleep on his bed is usually either very attached to it or has a dog with a very dominant position in the household. The question can also yield information about factors in the home environment which are helping to maintain the problem behaviour. For example, it may be useful to know whether or not (a) the dog is walked regularly, (b) whether it is left for long periods on its own, or (c) whether it follows the owner from room to room when he is at home. Eating arrangements can also be interesting, as the following example shows:

CASE EXAMPLE 8:1

Mr. and Mrs. A., a young couple without children, sought advice about Andy, a 3 year old male old English sheepdog. The chief problems were that he sometimes barred their way into the kitchen and he refused to come out of the car at the end of a journey. In both situations he would growl and snap, forcing the owners to retreat. When they talked about the rest of their life with Andy, it became clear that they had allowed him to become dominant by rewarding various dominant behaviours. The most striking instance occurred every morning. They had been concerned that the dog was not eating enough, so each morning Mr. A. had prepared a plate of cornflakes and milk, as if for himself, put it on the floor and pretended to start to eat it. Andy, stimulated by the competition, had come up and started eating as well, whereupon Mr. A. had withdrawn. This daily ritual had, of course, been extremely effective in teaching the dog dominance.

iii. **What is the composition of the household?**

This can yield important diagnostic clues. For example, if the household consists only of dog and owner, the dog's behaviour is probably greatly influenced by that of the owner and the owner may be very attached to the dog. If there are several small children in the house, the dog is unlikely to receive the owner's undivided attention for long. This may give rise to problems due to failure to observe and respond to the dog's behaviour (e.g. during housetraining). Also, it is often unrealistic to expect the mother of small children to carry out a time-consuming behaviour modification programme.

iv. **What is the relationship of the dog with other members of the household?**

Is it attached exclusively to the owner or is it attached to all family members? If it shows dominance aggression, does it do so towards all or just some family members? Are there some family members who are indifferent to, or actively dislike, the dog? Although it is rare for the whole family to attend a consultation and often other members are reported to be sceptical about the whole venture, the treatment of many problems requires at least some co-operation on their part.

It is also important to know about the dog's relationship with other dogs in the household, especially the dominance relationships between the various dogs; the owner's opinion as to which is 'top dog' should not be accepted without enquiring in more detail about the dogs' behaviour (see Chapter 9.8).

v. **What is the owner's attitude towards the dog and towards its problem?**

The owner's general attitude towards his dog is something which is best not elicited by direct questioning, but usually emerges when covering the areas outlined above. On the other hand, direct questions can often be fruitfully asked about the owner's attitude towards the problem behaviour. This is important for two reasons. Firstly, owners usually have their own theories about the dog's behaviour; they often misinterpret it in ways which cause extra distress to themselves and the dog. It is important to elicit these misconceptions so that they can be corrected. Secondly, it is important to know how willing the owner is to tolerate the behaviour, as this has a bearing on treatment. If the owner is at his wit's end, with the possibility of euthanasia not far away, a plan of treatment might be adopted which is likely to yield quick, dramatic results, but with some risk of side effects; this could be a situation where the careful use of punishment might be indicated or medication might of be prescribed. On the other hand, if the owner is prepared to tolerate the behaviour a little longer, a purely behavioural approach, based on extinction of the undesirable behaviour and rewarding alternative desirable responses, would be indicated.

FORMULATING AN EXPLANATION

8.3. INTERPRETATION OF THE BEHAVIOUR

In formulating an explanation of the problem, it is often first helpful to try to make sense of the dog's behaviour, using the following conceptual scheme:

a.   **Is what the dog is doing part of a sequence of instinctive behaviour?**

Clues to this are normally to be found (a) in the details of the dog's bodily posture, vocalisation etc. as he engages in the behaviour (b) in the context in which the behaviour occurs (c) in the behaviour of the dog at other times. One of the most common instinctive behaviour sequences involved in problem behaviour is dominance aggression; sexual, predatory and fear-induced behaviour are other examples.

EXAMPLE

A dog barks when the door bell rings. Is this protective aggression or something else, e.g. excitement at an impending social occasion? The behaviour is more likely to be protective aggression if: (a) the dog growls as well as barking (b) the barking is more intense when strangers approach the house than when habitual visitors do so (c) the dog shows other territorial behaviour, e.g. it barks at passers-by when left alone in the car.

b.   **Is there a learned component in the behaviour?**

This should be suspected if the behaviour is rewarded, even only some of the time. Experiences which commonly reward problem behaviour are the owner's attention (even though it is unfavourable) and new, interesting sights and sounds (see Chapter 3.2).

c.   **Is the behaviour influenced by anxiety or over-excitement?**

This should be suspected if

i.   the dog's problem behaviour has motor or autonomic components which are signs of high arousal, e.g. restlessness, displacement activities, trembling, urinating, attempting to escape;

ii.   the dog seems generally over-anxious or over-aroused;

iii.   the problem behaviour occurs in a situation which typically causes anxiety in dogs (e.g. separation from owner);

iv.   there are conditions in the dog's environment which might be expected to cause a state of anxiety (e.g. frequent or inconsistent punishment, family conflicts, neurotic owner, adverse early experiences).

It should be borne in mind that these possible explanations of the dog's behaviour are not mutually exclusive. It can have both instinctive and learned components as well as being exacerbated by anxiety.

8.4. CAUSATION

Having made some sense of the behaviour, as far as possible the following questions about causation should be answered:

a.   **Is the behaviour influenced by hormonal factors?**

This should be suspected if the problem behaviour is related to sexual behaviour (e.g. roaming, mounting or territory-marking) or to dominance aggression. It should also be suspected if the problem started or recurs around times of presumed hormonal change (e.g. puberty, full maturity, oestrus, after spaying); this can give a clue to the hormonal origin of behaviour whose causation otherwise appears obscure.

CASE EXAMPLE 8:2

Mrs. G. sought treatment for Gemma, a 12 year-old Labrador retriever bitch who had recently started to destroy furniture on a horrendous scale when left alone in the house; she had already disembowelled two mattresses and a sofa. She also destroyed her bedding when left alone in the kitchen at night. The behaviour was suggestive of the typical instinctive response of a dog suffering from separation anxiety (see Chapter 10), as it only occurred when the dog could not gain access to the owners. It was not clear, however, why she should start to respond in this way at this time in her life. Gemma had previously been a placid family pet and had always been accustomed to being left for hours alone in the house during the day. It emerged during the consultation that the behaviour had started soon after the dog had been spayed, following a pyrometra. It seemed possible, therefore, that hormonal factors were influencing the behaviour: that it was due, perhaps, to a decrease in progestagen production as a result of spaying. Gemma was treated for a month with megestrol acetate (Ovarid, Coopers Pitman-Moore). Three days after the first administration of the drug all destructive tendencies ceased.

b. **Is the behaviour influenced by genetic or constitutional factors or early environment?**

Genetic factors should be suspected if it is a typical behaviour for the breed (e.g. sudden aggression in whole-colour cocker spaniels, fear of noises in Border collies) or if there is evidence that either parent showed the same behaviour. Early environment may be implicated if there is evidence of the appropriate adverse experiences (see Chapter 6.2). Any of the three factors (genetic, constitutional or environmental) may be responsible if the dog has always shown the behaviour. If any of these three factors are operating, the amount of improvement which can be achieved is more limited, although some constitutionally based disorders, such as hyperactivity, improve with age.

c. **What are the stimuli which trigger the behaviour?**

The more precisely these can be defined, the more effective behavioural treatment will be. Relevant stimuli can include place, time of day, owner behaviour, presence or absence of other people or dogs and the occurrence of certain smells or sounds.

d. **How does the problem behaviour relate to the rest of the dog's behaviour?**

Are there certain general tendencies (such as dominance or hyperactivity) which should be tackled before the specific problem can be dealt with?

e. **Is the owner's attitude contributing to the problem?**

If so, some attempt will have to be made to modify the attitude.

TREATMENT

The general principles of behavioural treatment based on learning theory have been discussed in Chapter 3. Before discussing how to formulate a treatment plan it is appropriate to discuss here the general principles of surgical and psychopharmacological methods of treatment.

8.5. SURGICAL TREATMENT

Attempts are sometimes made to treat behaviour problems by removing part of the body so that the dog is physically unable to engage in the behaviour: for example by removing the canine teeth of biting dogs or the tails of tail-chasers. Tail-chasing is rarely cured by tail removal, the dog continuing to chase the stump. It is reported (Houpt & Wolski, 1982) that aggressive dogs whose teeth are removed, as well as being unable to inflict as much damage, often become less aggressive, presumably because their owners feel more confident in standing up to them or because they learn that biting achieves less satisfactory results. Veterinary surgeons, however, are often understandably unwilling to mutilate a dog in this way. **Castration** is the operation most often performed for behavioural reasons, usually because of gender-related behaviour problems such as intermale aggression, mounting, roaming and urine-marking. However, the evidence is that the effect of castration on these responses is variable, ranging from 90% in roaming to 50-60% in urine marking, mounting and aggression (Hopkins *et al* 1976). The age of the dog is not a good predictor of its response to castration. Castration is ineffective in such a high proportion of cases probably because (a) the male brain is perinatally affected by higher levels of testosterone secretion (Hart & Ladewig, 1979), and (b) learning is also involved in the behaviour, which may continue out of habit.

Spaying of bitches is sometimes undertaken for a variety of behavioural reasons. There is no evidence, however, that spaying has a beneficial effect on any behaviour other than that related directly to oestrus and false pregnancies. A study by O'Farrell and Peachey (1990) found that when the change in behaviour of 150 spayed bitches pre-operatively and 6 months post-operatively was compared with the change in unspayed controls, the spayed bitches showed a significant increase in two kinds of behaviour:

a. indiscriminate appetite: this behaviour is presumably connected with weight gain;

b. dominance aggression towards family members.

The bitches in the spayed group mostly responsible for this difference were puppies under one year already showing some aggression. Of these, in the spayed group, half became more aggressive and half improved. In the unspayed group, only 14% got worse and 86% improved. The practical implication of these findings seems to be that, if possible, it would be better at least to postpone spaying of these aggressive puppies until their behaviour has improved.

All these surgical procedures have the disadvantage that they are irreversible. If they are seriously contemplated, where possible their probable effects should first be tested pharmacologically. With castration, this is possible using delmadinone (Tardak, Syntex).

Any attempt to alter behaviour by surgical means should always be immediately followed by behavioural treatment; there is otherwise a much higher risk of the undesirable behaviour continuing or reappearing.

8.6. DRUG TREATMENT

Specialists in animal behaviour problems differ in the extent to which they use drugs. Understandably, veterinary surgeons are among the more frequently users. In general, the benefits of using drugs are that:

a. Some cases respond dramatically to medication: this can be of critical importance when the problem is severe and/or the owner is at the end of his tether.

b. In some cases, there is also a placebo effect on the owner. For example, a treatment programme which includes medication may seem more credible to him and he may be more motivated to carry it out.

The disadvantages are:

a. Some drugs (e.g. megestrol) are expensive in the doses needed to treat large dogs.

b.   There is a risk of undesirable side effects (e.g. adrenal suppression with megestrol) or paradoxical effects (e.g. over-excitement induced by diazepam).

c.   Most drugs can be given only for a short time in most cases because over time there is an increased risk of side effects (megestrol) or because habituation is likely to occur (diazepam). They therefore cannot on their own change behaviour permanently: they can only alter the dog's mood state in a way which facilitates the learning of new behaviour patterns. Thus, permanent change can only result from behavioural treatment.

d.   There is, therefore, a danger that when medication is used, both specialist and client place undue reliance upon it and neglect behavioural treatment.

In general it is best to reserve the use of medication for cases which are serious, at crisis point or where medication is necessary to obtain client cooperation. **Drugs should never be used without concurrent behavioural treatment.**

At the moment there are few drugs licensed for the treatment of behaviour disorders in small animals; these are mainly sedatives or synthetic progestagens. By contrast, a wide range of drugs is available for psychiatric treatment of human beings. Many of these (e.g. diazepam) have been used in experimental situations with animals, but there have been few clinical trials: for the most part, recommendations are based on clinical impressions.

Tranquillisers

Acepromazine maleate (Acetylpromazine, C-Vet) may be used to reduce anxiety or excitability. Its disadvantages are that it may produce excessive sedation and that there is a risk of cardiovascular side effects if it is used over a long period. As alternatives, two groups of drugs not licensed for animal use, the benzodiazepines, especially diazepam (Valium, Roche), and the tricyclic antidepressants [e.g. amitriptyline (Tryptizol, Morson)] have been used successfully. With these drugs also, it may be difficult to find a dosage which relieves anxiety or reduces excitement without causing undue sedation; the distance in terms of comparative dosage between the two thresholds is much less in dogs than it is in human beings. As a starting point, a dosage of 2 mg/kg before the anxiety provoking event has been recommended for diazepam and of 2—4 mg/kg for amitriptyline (Voith, 1984). With diazepam, paradoxical effects, such as hyperactivity, have been reported. Because of the risk of side effects from any drug not licensed for animal use, a dog should not be left unattended for the first twenty-four hours of regular administration of the drug.

Because of the possibility that such drugs may inhibit learning, they should only be used when the dog is so anxious that effective behavioural treatment cannot otherwise be embarked on. In addition, when the drug is used and behavioural treatment is successful, it is possible that the dog may learn to be calm in a certain situation when under the influence of the drug but may not generalise its learning to the undrugged state. After successful treatment, therefore, the drug should be withdrawn in gradual stages.

Synthetic progestagens

Of the synthetic progestagens, megestrol acetate (Ovarid, Coopers Pitman-Moore) is the most widely used for treatment of behaviour problems. It is most clearly indicated as an adjunct to the treatment of gender-related problem behaviour such as dominance aggression, mounting, roaming and urine-marking. It also has more general effects on the central nervous system, tending to make dogs more tractable and more equable in mood. This makes the drug effective in a wider range of disorders, such as destructiveness, where emotionality or over-arousal are contributing factors. A starting dose of 2 mg/kg daily for two weeks is recommended, followed by half that dose for a further two weeks.

If the initial dose is ineffective, a dose of 4 mg/kg can be tried. **As with other physical treatments, the administration of megestrol should always be accompanied by behavioural treatment.** The drug should be regarded as a means for providing the optimum conditions for behavioural treatment to take effect. As it cannot safely be administered on a long-term basis, it cannot be regarded as a treatment in itself. A study by Joby *et al* (1984) found an initial improvement rate of 75% after two — four weeks in male dogs treated for a range of behavioural disorders with megestrol alone, but adequate data on the long term follow-up of such cases are not available.

Some dogs respond dramatically to megestrol and relapse when it is withdrawn, despite the owner's best efforts with behavioural treatment. In these cases, the course of medication may be repeated after 3 months, by which time adrenal function is likely to have returned to normal levels (Van den Broek, personal communication). Where appropriate, a safer (but possibly less effective) alternative would be delmadinone as a prelude to possible castration (see previous section).

Opioid antagonists

Recently these have been found to be useful in the treatment of stereotypies (Chapter 10.6).

8.7. DIET

At the moment the topic of diet and its effect on behaviour is as controversial in the case of dogs as it is with people. Some animal behaviourists recommend a change of diet almost routinely, while others consider that diet affects behaviour only rarely. There are plenty of case reports of dramatic improvement in behaviour following a change in diet, but as yet no controlled studies. The mechanisms most often postulated for such an effect are an allergic response to some component of the diet or an intolerance of high levels of protein or of low quality protein.

Given the present state of knowledge, it may be worth trying an experimental change of diet in cases where the problem involves the dog's general behaviour rather than behaviour in a specific situation, especially if:

a.   the behaviour seems peculiar and not fully explicable in other terms.

b.   there are also physical signs of allergy or food intolerance.

c.   there was a change of diet around the time of the onset of the behaviour problem.

d.   the dog's present diet is nutritionally inappropriate (e.g. all meat).

A test diet of one part lamb to four parts boiled rice (wet weight) covers the possibilities of allergic response and protein intolerance.

8.8. BEHAVIOURAL TREATMENT

A different programme of behavioural treatment must be formulated for each individual case but, in doing so, the following conceptual framework may be useful:

Are alterations needed in the dog's general behavioural disposition? The alterations most commonly required are:

i. Establishment of owner dominance

This is most obviously necessary when the dog is showing aggression towards family members (Chapter 9.2). It is often also necessary when the dog shows other types of aggression towards people or other dogs (Chapter 9.3,4,6,7,8). In addition, there are other behaviour problems which do not involve aggression but which can be improved by increasing owner dominance. The most obvious example is a problem which involves poor response to the owner's commands. However, many cases in which the dog is showing signs of dominance over the owner (independent life style and/or frequently making demands on the owner or taking the social initiative) may benefit from increasing owner dominance, even though there is no obvious relation between the specific problem and dominance. Methods of establishing owner dominance are described in Chapter 9.2.

ii. Reduction of stress

This should be attempted for dogs with general disorders of emotionality, either general anxiety, over-excitement or destructiveness in the owner's absence (see Chapter 10). Whatever the problem, it should also be attempted when there is evidence that the dog is being subjected to abnormal stress: if, for example:

a. it is being constantly punished;

b. it is likely to find its life confusing or unpredictable, either because its owner behaves inconsistently towards it, because different family members reward or punish different behaviour or because the general family situation is tense or chaotic;

c. it has recently been rehomed.

Methods of reducing stress are outlined in Chapter 10.

To tackle the specific problem:

i. Removal or alteration of triggering stimuli

In most cases, it is worth starting by attempting to remove or alter the stimulus which elicits the problem behaviour, so that, if successful, the behaviour disappears. Then:

a. in a few cases this may be all that is needed. For example, a dog which growls and snaps when it is groomed might be taken to a professional groomer or its coat might be cut short; a dog which urinates at night when shut in the kitchen might be allowed access to the owner's bedroom. These are methods of managing rather than solving problems and the aim of most behavioural consultations is to find solutions to replace such management methods. In some cases, however, they may be appropriate: for example, if the triggering stimulus is an unnecessary feature of the dog's life; if the owners are unwilling or unable to undertake more complex behavioural treatment; if the dog is old and infirm. (It should be noted, however, that age *per se* is not a contra-indication for behaviour modification.)

b. In most cases, it is not enough to remove or alter the triggering stimulus, either because it is necessary to the dog's or the owner's life or because the problem behaviour will reappear in response to new stimuli: for example, excitement and barking in response to the telephone ringing may be temporarily eliminated by changing the sound of the ring, but it will usually reappear when the dog learns the meaning of the new sound. It is, therefore, necessary to break the connection between the triggering stimulus and the undesirable response. Broadly speaking, the methods of doing this (which are complementary rather than mutually exclusive) are as follows:

i. Extinction

The rewards for the undesirable behaviour are removed e.g. a dog which pesters the family for tit-bits at meal times is ignored. This will not work on its own when the behaviour itself is enjoyable or self-rewarding, e.g. barking.

ii   **Response substitution**

The dog is taught to respond to the triggering stimulus with an acceptable action rather with the undesirable behaviour. For example, a dog might learn to sit in the hall when the bell rings rather than running to the door barking. This learning will take place more easily if:

a.   The dog first of all learns the alternative response in circumstances where there are no competing responses (e.g. the dog is taught to sit in the hall when there is no door bell ringing).

b.   The dog is highly motivated to perform the alternative response because

   i) The response obtains an attractive reward. The attractiveness of a reward can be enhanced by being made a secondary as well as a primary reinforcer (see Chapter 3.10). Thus, the dog might be rewarded for sitting in the hall with a toy which had previously been associated with enjoyable play sessions.

   ii) The response is itself intrinsically enjoyable: responses which are motivated by the same instinct which prompts the instinctive behaviour have an advantage (e.g. chasing a ball as an alternative to chasing sheep).

iii)   **Systematic desensitization**

Usually this refers to a method of treating anxiety whereby the dog in a non-anxious state is presented with a version of the triggering stimulus which does not provoke anxiety: starting with a very mild stimulus, the intensity of the stimulus can be gradually increased as treatment progresses (Chapter 10.2). However, the method can also be applied to problems in which other states of high arousal are involved e.g. excitement, aggression. In essence, the method consists of response substitution (see ii. above), plus presentation of the triggering stimulus in gradually increasing degrees of intensity. Thus, the dog which barks at visitors is taught its sitting-in-the-hall routine first of all when no visitors are in the offing; the next step might be to have it sit while a visitor approaches the door and goes away without ringing the bell and so on.

iv.   **Distraction**

The dog is prevented from responding to the triggering stimulus by distracting it with a startling (and sometimes unpleasant) stimulus. The effectiveness of this method is greatly increased if it is combined with response substitution. The effectiveness of the startling stimulus can be increased by pre-conditioning it: giving it a negative connotation by associating it with an unpleasant or frustrating experience (see Chapter 3.11). Care should be taken not to upset or frighten the dog excessively as this may lead to behavioural side-effects such as fear or aggression. In cases where the problem is caused by anxiety or stress, the distracting stimulus must be so mild as not to upset or frighten the dog at all.

8.9.   OWNER'S ATTITUDES AND RELATED FACTORS

The successful treatment of a behaviour problem in a dog usually involves a change in the owner's behaviour as well as that of the dog. Treatment plans which are theoretically correct from the point of view of the dog's behaviour frequently fail because the owner does not carry them out. It is, therefore, worth devoting attention to the factors which might facilitate or hinder a change of behaviour on the part of the owner.

a.   **Objective circumstances**

Sometimes an owner simply cannot carry out a particular behavioural programme because of domestic or work commitments. It is better to be aware of an owner's limitations in this regard from the outset, so that he does not feel he is required to do the impossible.

b. **Mistaken ideas about dog psychology**

Correcting an owner's misinterpretations of his dog's behaviour is often an important prerequisite of change. For example, an owner may see his dog's destructiveness or aggression in a moral light, which may upset him or lead to the inappropriate use of punishment. It is worth taking trouble to ensure that he has understood the correct interpretation of the behaviour.

c. **The owner's attitude towards his dog**

The psychological function of the dog for the owner often plays a part in the development and maintenance of problem behaviour (see Chapter 7.4 for details of methods of modifying owner attitudes). Sometimes owners can be induced to modify these attitudes, either by gaining some insight into them or as a result of carrying out a behavioural programme (see Chapter 7.6). However, frequently the attitude must just be accepted and taken into account both in drawing up a plan of treatment and in presenting it to the client. For example, there is no point trying to urge the owner of a dog which urinates in the kitchen during the night out of separation distress to let it into the bedroom if the owner is horrified by the idea of dogs in bedrooms. She might find a regime of getting up in the middle of the night before the time the dog customarily urinates more acceptable. Similarly, when an extremely attached owner of a dominant dog is being urged to ignore it most of the time to re-establish owner dominance, it is often wise to present this regime as a temporary one which can be relaxed once dominance is established. Otherwise, the owner might find the regime quite unacceptable; as one owner asked plaintively, "Can't I even give him his good-night kiss?"

The owner's readiness to alter his attitude towards his dog and his view of his dog's behaviour is often the crucial factor in determining the success of a treatment. The owner, of course, can potentially observe much more of the dog's behaviour and his own behaviour towards the dog than can the clinician. If he can be encouraged to stand back and do this in the light of the new conceptual framework suggested to him, the potential for change is enormously increased. **The most successful treatment procedures are often not those carried out blindly by the owner on the instructions of the clinician, but those which are correctly modified and extended by the owner in the light of the new concepts the clinician has provided.**

Conversely, where the owner is unable to understand or accept the principles on which treatment is based, success is much less likely in the long term, especially if the dog has permanent personality attributes (such as dominance or excitability) which must be controlled because they cannot be cured.

CASE EXAMPLE 8:3.

Mr. and Mrs. C., a middle aged couple, sought treatment for a four year-old Border collie named Captain. The referral was precipitated by the dog biting the postman. The postman had been angry and said he would inform the police. The couple were very frightened, dreading that a policeman would appear on the doorstep to take away and destroy the dog. It emerged that this incident could have been predicted. The dog had been showing marked protective aggression for some time. He spent much of his time at a large picture window in the sitting room watching the passers-by in the street and visitors approaching the house, barking ferociously at those to which he objected. If allowed into the front garden he would make threatening forays into the street and when being walked on the lead he would sometimes lunge at passers-by. Although the dog had never bitten any of the family, he otherwise showed behaviour typical of a dominant dog, living an independent life and initiating most social interactions (see Chapter 9.2). It was recommended that the protective aggression be treated by initially keeping Captain away from situations which provoked him, such as the sitting-room window, until the owners had established more dominance over him. He was then to be gradually re-exposed to these situations, under the owners' control, with quiet non-aggressive behaviour being rewarded. Megestrol was also prescribed. An attempt was made to explain to the owners that, unless the dog's position of dominance in the household was reversed and unless they predicted and controlled his behaviour to some extent, rather than passively watching to see what he would do next, the protective aggression would continue.

When Mr. and Mrs. C. were seen two weeks later they reported some improvement. Enquiry into details, however, suggested that although they had carried out some of the instructions, they did not fully understand their rationale. The police had not taken up the matter of the bitten postman and it seemed that, the immediate crisis having been resolved, they did not want to give the matter much further thought.

A follow-up one year later, by a student for teaching purposes, confirmed this impression. There had been no further potential police involvement and the owners seemed to accept Captain's behaviour, talking indulgently about his 'naughtiness'. However, he still continued to bark at the window and threaten passers-by in the street. In conversation, the student gained the impression that Mr. and Mrs. C. had completely forgotten any instructions about establishing and maintaining dominance.

When dealing with an owner in whom a change of attitude is hard to bring about, a veterinary surgeon has an advantage over a specialist consultant, in that in most cases he maintains a relationship with a client over a longer period. He thus has an opportunity to repeat and reinforce ideas which the client finds difficult to accept.

8.10. ALTERNATIVES TO TREATMENT

It must be borne in mind that the improvement of quality of life of the whole family in which the dog lives is the primary purpose of a consultation. When the matter is viewed from this perspective, it is sometimes wiser not to attempt to treat the behaviour disorder, but to recommend **euthanasia**. The conditions which should suggest such a decision are that (a) the dog is so dangerous that it would present an unacceptable hazard even if it engaged in the problem behaviour only rarely (b) there is no way of telling whether the problem behaviour has been eliminated, other than waiting to see whether it is repeated. A household with young children who have already been severely bitten is the example of this situation most often encountered. Young children are particularly at risk because they cannot be reliably taught to understand the dog's body language and thus avoid attack. Another situation in which these conditions might apply is where the dog's aggression is so explosive and unpredictable that even adult owners continue to be at risk.

There are also some situations in which the best option seems to be to recommend that the owner try to **find another home for the dog**. Although on the whole it is probably inadvisable to encourage the re-cycling of dogs with behavioural problems, there are cases in which the dog's particular domestic situation or the personality of the owner seems to be making such a large contribution to the problem that this solution is justified. In these circumstances, breed rescue societies are often helpful in finding new homes for these dogs.

CASE EXAMPLE: 8:4

A widow in her sixties brought two cavalier King Charles spaniels aged one year; her complaint was that they barked uncontrollably when they heard an unusual noise or when visitors approached the house. It emerged that she lived in a council house and that the terms of the lease forbade her to keep any pets. The neighbours had complained about the barking and had eventually reported the dogs to the council, which had ordered her to get rid of them. In fact, she had five dogs altogether, but the council did not know about the other three. She felt so strongly about the whole matter that she was contemplating buying another house in which she could live unmolested with all her dogs. Her daughter, who accompanied her, indicated that such a plan was not realistic. She also said her mother suffered from a severe heart complaint which made it hard for her to manage and exercise so many dogs. In this situation, the best solution seemed to be to prevail on the owner to find a new home for the two youngest dogs. As they were young and pure-bred, there seemed to be a good prospect of finding suitable new homes for them. In addition, if each were found separate homes with no other dogs, it seemed likely that the barking could be brought under control. The daughter welcomed these recommendations with enthusiasm and the owner said she would consider them. Unfortunately, there is no follow-up information available on this case.

There are some cases where the prognosis seems poor, but where the owners are keen to attempt treatment. In these instances it is often advisable to comply with this wish, for two reasons:

a.   In the present state of knowledge it is not possible to predict the outcome of treatment with anything approaching certainty;

b.   even when treatment fails and the animal has to be destroyed, an owner can often make this decision with greater peace of mind knowing that he has tried everything.

FURTHER READING

MARDER, A.R. (1991). Psychotropic drugs and behavioural therapy. *The Veterinary Clinic of North America,* 21, 329-342.

FURTHER READING FOR OWNERS

NEVILLE, P. (1991). Do Dogs Need Shrinks? Sidgwick & Jackson.

O'FARRELL, V. (1989) Problem Dog: Behaviour or Misbehaviour. Methuen, London.

Table 1
Diagnosis and treatment of behaviour problems: Summary

Description of problem

What exactly does
dog do?

When and where does
it do it?

What happens afterwards?

History

When did behaviour start?

In what circumstances
did it start?

Treatment methods
already tried

General information

Rest of dog's behaviour
Dog's daily routine
Composition of household
Relationship of dog to
other family members
Owner's attitudes

Interpretation of the behaviour

Which aspects are instinctive?

Which aspects are learned?

Is anxiety or over-excitement involved?

Causation

Are hormonal factors involved?

Are there genetic, constitutional or early environmental factors?

What are the triggering stimuli?

How does the problem relate to the rest of the dog's behaviour?

Is the owner's attitude a contributing factor?

Treatment methods available
Surgical: Castration

Drugs
Tranquillisers
Synthetic progestagens

Behavioural:
General
Establishment of owner dominance
Reduction of stress

Specific
Removal or alteration of triggering stimulus
Extinction
Response substitution
Systematic desensitization
Distraction

Modification of owner attitudes
Altering the cognitive component
Altering the behavioural component
Facilitating insight.

TREATMENT OF AGGRESSION

Chapter Nine_____

Predatory aggression; defensive aggression: dominance aggression; possessive aggression; protective aggression; fear-induced aggression; noise provoked aggression; 'rage' syndrome; maternal aggression; aggression directed towards other dogs

Aggression is the commonest problem encountered in behavioural practice. In dogs, it may be directed towards people, towards other dogs, towards some other species such as sheep or cats or towards objects such as cars, bicycles or telephones.

The first distinction to be made when assessing a case showing aggression is between defensive aggression and predatory aggression.

9.1. PREDATORY AGGRESSION

This may be directed towards any kind of animal, including dogs and human beings. It may even be directed towards inanimate objects such as cars or bicycles. It is typical of predatory aggression that it is elicited by quarry which run or move quickly. It is also typical that when the dog reaches the quarry it does not growl, threaten or attempt to communicate with it in any way. In the most straightforward case it will attack the quarry until it is motionless (i.e. presumed to be dead). That dogs often abandon this aim before it is achieved (e.g. chase sheep for a short distance and then turn back) is probably due to the fact that the stimulus is not strong enough to elicit the chasing behaviour in its full form in that particular dog. Quite frequently, however, the dog will stop a short distance from the quarry and bark. This is probably because, when viewed at close quarters, there are certain aspects of the quarry which inhibit attack; it may present an anatomical puzzle (e.g. if it is a bicycle) or it may look too fierce and threatening (e.g. a cat which turns and hisses). The barking here is displacement activity produced by conflict (see Chapter 5.4).

DIAGNOSIS

Predatory aggression against dogs

Typically the attack is preceded by a chase, triggered by the victim running. It is most often shown by larger dogs towards smaller dogs and by breeds which are bred for this behaviour, such as greyhounds.

Predatory aggression directed against human beings

This is rarely directed towards adults in its most complete and dangerous form, although cases in the USA have been described (Beck & Voith, 1983) where adults or adolescents have been killed by dogs showing predatory aggression. In most of these cases more than one dog was involved and the dogs had been aroused just before the attack by chasing some other quarry which had unexpectedly disappeared. There is evidence that the victim triggered the attack by moving or running; in some instances victims survived because they lay down and did not move, causing the dogs to abandon the attack.

Usually, however, cases of predatory aggression towards adults are less serious. A new form which has emerged in recent years is chasing joggers.

Predatory aggression against infants is more often dangerous. Typically, the dog is not familiar with babies, only with adults or older children. Presumably the attacks are triggered by movements or sounds made by the babies. As with predatory attacks on other species, a baby who is safe in one situation (say, in a pram) may be at risk in another (for example, lying on the floor). **New parents whose dog is unfamiliar with babies should, therefore, monitor its behaviour in a range of situations before being satisfied that it is safe with the baby.**

Predatory attacks on other species

A whole range of live creatures and inanimate objects can become the victims of predatory attack. Small animals such as rabbits, birds and cats are commonly recognised targets. Owners and society generally tend to accept this aspect of dogs' behaviour. Owners can be taken by surprise, however, when the attack is directed at a household pet with whom the dog has lived harmoniously up to this point. For example, a cat or rabbit which is normally treated with courtesy may be chased when it is glimpsed running in the garden. Predatory aggression against livestock (for instance sheep) is another recognisable but, in this instance, quite unacceptable form of behaviour. The same activity may be directed towards moving machines, most commonly bicycles and cars. Typically the dog barks when it gets near the vehicle, presumably as a displacement activity because it does not see how to attack it.

TREATMENT

Predatory aggression is difficult to treat because

a.   it often involves victims such as animals and young children whose own behaviour is difficult to alter;

b.   it is an instinctive behaviour pattern which carries its own inbuilt reward; dogs will persist in chasing birds and rabbits even if they never catch any;

c.   in many instances the effect of the behaviour is so disastrous that treatment has failed if it occurs again on even one occasion.

A combination of the following methods may be tried:

a.   **Increasing the dominance and control of the owner over the dog**

This is often appropriate if the chasing occurs when the owner is present, especially if he reports that he calls the dog back but it does not respond. Often it emerges that the owner has poor dominance over the dog generally. In this case, treatment for dominance aggression as outlined in 9.2 is indicated. The owner should also practice repeatedly calling the dog to him, using a long rope or extending lead, first in circumstances where the dog is likely to respond, then in circumstances which are increasingly more exciting and likely to tempt the dog away. The dog should always be rewarded when it comes. It should be emphasised to the owner that he has the best chance of recalling the dog before it has seen the prey or, failing that, when it has seen the prey but has not started to run. This may seem obvious, but some owners become paralysed in the face of what they feel to be an inevitable chain of events.

b. Desensitization

The prey can be regarded as a stimulus which causes arousal. The aim of treatment then becomes to teach the dog to be calm in the presence of this previously arousing stimulus. The dog is put on an extending lead, which allows the owner to control it if need be, without the dog feeling restrained all the time. The treatment should start with some version of the prey which is unlikely to cause great excitement (e.g. a sheep lying down or a sleeping cat some distance away). The owner then brings the dog to the required distance from the stimulus, gets it to sit, praises it and feeds it tit-bits as long as it remains calm. The procedure is repeated, gradually increasing the excitement value of the stimulus, with several trials at each level. The excitement might be increased by the prey being nearer, moving increasingly quickly or consisting of a group of animals (e.g. a flock of sheep) rather than just one. If at any point the dog shows any excitement, it is told sharply 'No' and all forms of reward are immediately stopped. The treatment then continues at a lower level of excitement. Over the period when this treatment is carried out, care should be taken not to expose the dog in its everyday life to more exciting versions of the stimulus.

The drawback of this approach is that it demands some ingenuity and considerable dedication on the part of the owner.

c. Punishment

This is one of the situations in which punishing the behaviour may be an effective way of eliminating it, especially if the dog is of otherwise stable personality (see Chapter 3.11). Sheep-chasing is the problem for which shock collars are most often used, reportedly with success, but the risk of using such a device must be borne in mind (see Chapter 3.12). It is often possible, with some ingenuity, to devise less dangerous aversive stimuli. There are two points in the chasing sequence at which the aversive stimulus is likely to be most effective, depending on circumstances. The first is when the dog first catches sight of the prey, before its excitement has had time to rise. The owner intervenes with a startling or distracting stimulus (e.g. rape alarm, training disks) and then immediately substitutes an alternative response which is rewarded. In these circumstances, the most attractive alternative response is often that of chasing another moving object such as a ball (preferably kept especially for this purpose and previously pre-conditioned as a secondary reinforcer (see Chapter 3.10)). Alternatively, the aversive stimulus can be applied as the dog approaches the victim: this is most likely to be effective when the victim himself produces the stimulus (e.g. suddenly opened umbrella, bucket of water, rape alarm) but the stimulus may have to be stronger and more startling, because the dog may be more excited at this point in the chase.

This approach may be more effective if a desensitization hierachy of victims can be arranged i.e. starting with only mildly interesting victims and proceeding gradually to more exciting ones.

PREVENTION

Like most problems, predatory aggression is easier to prevent than to cure. Pet dogs should not be encouraged to chase prey of any kind. When young they should also be positively taught not to chase various kinds of animal (e.g. sheep) by leading them past the animal repeatedly: if the puppy shows interest, it should be distracted and an acceptable response substituted.

DEFENSIVE AGGRESSION

This can be classified according to the kind of threat which elicits it.

9.2 DOMINANCE AGGRESSION

Here the perceived threat is a social one: a challenge to the dog's dominant status. It is, therefore, only directed towards species (usually people or other dogs) which the dog assumes will understand his body language (see Chapter 4.1). Dominance aggression towards other dogs is dealt with in 9.8.

DIAGNOSIS

The manifestation of dominance aggression towards people which most commonly drives owners to seek advice is biting or growling. Although the owner may sometimes report that the dog bites unpredictably or without provocation, questioning almost always reveals that there is a pattern to its attacks and that they are triggered by some stimulus. The aggression is usually provoked by actions by the victim which the dog perceives as threatening its dominance. Typically, the victim's actions fall into one or more of the following categories:

a. Patting or grooming the dog or touching its hindquarters.

b. Trying to take away food, a bone or some other object the dog has in its possession.

c. Invading a location the dog perceives to be its territory. The dog may be left there undisturbed for long periods of the day and comes to assume special rights over it. Typically, this can happen when a dog has been confined to the kitchen; the owners suddenly find that it will not let them in.

d. Disturbing the dog in its habitual resting place. It may show aggression if the owner tries to turn it off a chair or bed. Children may be bitten if they accidentally brush against the dog in its basket.

e. Giving the dog a command, particularly one which calls for a submissive action, such as sitting, lying or giving up something.

Although the owner may have been driven to seek help by aggression shown in one of these situations, the dog may show aggression in some of the others also, perhaps to a lesser extent. Frequently it displays a typical pattern of interaction with the owners; it may live a relatively independent life, not following the owners around all the time, but seeking company only at certain times and then often to make a specific request, such as to be let out. If it does choose to be in the owner's company all the time, the owner is the compliant recipient of its constant demands for attention: when these are denied, it becomes ever more insistent. Although it may not show aggression when given a command, it will often obey commands slowly or after several repetitions.

It may sometimes be hard to tell whether a dog reacts with aggression to a particular kind of event (e.g. being touched) because it perceives it as a dominance threat or out of fear (Chapter 9.5). However, each type of aggression is normally accompanied by a characteristic body posture (see Chapter 4.6 and Chapter 9.5). In addition, dominance aggression in a particular situation is normally accompanied by other kinds of dominant behaviour within the family. Aggression provoked by a veterinary procedure is frequently fear-induced aggression.

CAUSES

a. **Genetic factors**

    There is no doubt that inherited factors play a part in dominance aggression. In fact, the guarding breeds are to a certain extent selectively bred to show that behaviour.

b.   **Hormonal factors**

Dominance aggression is more common in male dogs (Borchelt, 1983) and also in spayed bitches (O'Farrell and Peachey, 1990). It is probable that in the male dogs the behaviour, is at least, in part determined by perinatal hormonal influences (Hart, 1985).

c.   **Composition of the household**

If there is more than one dog in the household, their own dominance hierarchy, which is to some extent determined by the sexes and relative sizes of the dogs, will influence the tendency of each dog to show dominance aggression towards human beings. The dog at the top of the dog dominance hierarchy is thereby encouraged to show dominance aggression towards the owners.

The ages and sexes of the human members of the household will also influence the dog's tendency to show dominance aggression. It is more difficult for children and women to dominate dogs. Also, if there is no human male in the household, there is a greater tendency for a male dog to see itself as forming a pair bond with the female owner (Chapter 4.5).

d.   **Behaviour of the owners**

Dogs showing dominance aggression have often been unwittingly encouraged by the owners to view themselves as dominant in the household. Owners may do this by

i.   allowing the dog to take the initiative in most interactions and by complying with most of the dog's requests;

ii.   allowing the dog frequently to assume dominant postures such as placing its paws on the owner's shoulders or sleeping on the owner's bed;

iii. reinforcing displays of dominance aggression by withdrawing or backing down;

iv.   allowing the dog to spend too much of its time separate from the human members of the family. This may allow a dog with dominant tendencies to develop an independent life-style. It may also give it the impression that it has special rights over the territory over which it spends its time.

e.   **Owner attitudes**

Owners who show the kind of behaviour outlined above often feel towards the dog as they would towards a human friend or child and derive pleasure from complying with the dog's requests. Often, such owners have a liberal rather than an authoritarian attitude towards relationships in general; they find it distasteful always to be ordering the dog about (Chapter 7.4).

TREATMENT

a.   For the time being, **until the owner has gained a certain degree of dominance over the dog, he should take care to avoid the situations which tend to provoke aggression** as every successful confrontation by the dog increases its dominance. This may mean denying the dog access to places where it tends to behave in a dominant way. It may mean giving up attempts to groom the dog for a while. It may involve ignoring some misdemeanours, if confrontation might provoke aggression. If the dog tends to be aggressive over food, or guards its food bowl, the owner should try feeding it in another room, from another dish. In general, it may be possible to avoid some aggressive incidents by changing locations; a dog which is impossible to groom in the living room may be amenable if put in the bath.

b. **As far as possible the owner should ignore the dog.** Although he should reduce the frequency of his social approaches to the dog (chatting to it, calling it, petting it and so on) it is particularly important that he ignore the dog's approaches to him. This is designed to have two effects. Firstly, by deprivation, it increases the incentive of the owner's attention as a reward. Secondly, as ignoring another animal is, in a dog's eyes, a dominant way to behave, it increases the owner's dominance status (Chapter 4.8). In addition, where the owner's previous behaviour towards the dog was related to his emotional attachment to it, this new mode of behaviour may have the beneficial effect of making the owner more detached and objective (Chapter 7.6).

c. **The owner should reward only submissive actions on the part of the dog.** The most useful actions in this context are submissive postures such as sitting or lying, taken up in obedience to the owner's command. The owner can use his own attention as a reward in this context. He can also use a range of rewarding experiences in the dog's life, such as being let into the garden, having a ball thrown or being given a meal. For example, if the dog whines to be let out, the owner would not respond at that point; a few minutes later he would call the dog to the door, tell it to sit and then open the door.

d. As far as possible, **the owner should not allow the dog to make up its own mind how to spend its time.** He should tell it to come with him, sit, stay in its bed, etc.

e. **The owner should not permit the dog to take up postures which it might regard as dominant.** In particular, he should not allow it to jump up (particularly if it is a big dog which puts its paws on the owner's shoulders), put paws or lie on the owner's lap, curl round his shoulders or sleep on his bed.

f. The owner should not engage in 'tug-of-war' games with the dog.

g. **A daily session of standard obedience training is useful** for two reasons.
    Firstly, it is a situation in which the owner is clearly dominant. Secondly, the more automatic are a dog's responses to commands, the better chance the owner has of controlling the dog by means of them. Some owners find that keeping a lead on the dog in the house has a similar effect; it makes the dog feel less dominant and it increases the degree of physical control the owner has over it.

h. **It is often useful to administer megestrol** (Ovarid, Coopers Pitman-Moore) at the same time as the owner is trying to gain behavioural dominance over the dog (Chapter 8.6). In most cases it makes the owner's task easier. It should be emphasised to him that the drug can only be given for a short time and that when it is being gradually withdrawn he must careful to maintain his behavioural dominance. In the longer term, castration may be helpful.

i. It has been reported (Mugford, 1987) that some dominant dogs become markedly less aggressive when fed a diet low in protein (see Chapter 8.7).

j. **When the owner has established a more dominant relationship with the dog, he should gradually reintroduce the situations in which the dog was previously aggressive, taking care not to provoke aggression again.** The sequence of situations used is similar to that employed in systematic desensitization (Chapter 10.1); the situations should be made progressively more similar to those which previously provoked aggression. Thus, if a dog was likely to bite when groomed, the owner could begin by patting the dog, praising it as long as it remains calm. He could then pat it with a brush in one hand, then groom it briefly on a relatively insensitive part of the body and so on. Before exposing the dog to these possibly provoking situations, the owner should emphasise his own dominant status to the dog, for example by giving it a command. In behaviour problems where dominance plays a part, an intervention by the owner **before** the provocative stimulus has two advantages: it distracts the dog and encourages an alternative, desirable response; it also reminds the dog of his subordinate position in the family hierarchy.

k. **Changing owner attitudes.** For many owners, explaining how a dog learns to be dominant and how the owners can reverse the process by their own behaviour is enough to produce a change in attitude. For some, however, it is necessary to direct efforts specifically towards persuading them to behave differently. It may be helpful to recommend the regime of ignoring the dog as a temporary one, which can be relaxed somewhat as the owner achieves dominance. It may also be useful to point out that they may well find the behaviour of the dog which results from the regime much more gratifying i.e. that the dog is likely to be more affectionate and less independent.

l. Sometimes the dog behaves in a dominant way towards certain members of the family only. One common pattern is that the husband is dominant over the dog, whereas the wife and children are not. Another less common pattern is that the dog is aggressive towards the husband but not the wife. It often turns out in this case that the wife has formed a special attachment to the dog, which comes to regard itself as having formed a pair bond with her; it then has the confidence constantly to challenge the husband for dominance. **Where the dog is selectively dominant within the family, the dominant family member should have nothing to do with the dog at all,** all rewards, including food, walks and social interaction being dispensed (according to the regime outlined above) by those to whom the dog had previously shown aggression.

It should be emphasised to owners that dominance aggression, like alcoholism in the view of Alcoholics Anonymous, is never cured; it can only be controlled. Owners must, therefore, always be on the watch for a further bid for dominance. In one series of 24 cases (Line & Voith, 1986) only 3 failed completely to respond to treatment but only one showed no aggression at all.

CASE EXAMPLE 9:1.

Mr. and Mrs. H., a married couple in their thirties, both teachers, sought advice about a fourteen year-old Cairn Terrier called Henry. They had teenage children and Henry had grown up with the family. He had recently developed the habit of growling and biting unexpectedly. Typically, he would approach a member of the family for attention. If she was sitting down he might climb on her knee. He would tolerate only a certain amount of patting and caressing, before suddenly turning and snapping. They were particularly alarmed when he did this to their four year-old niece. They had got to the point where they were almost hoping for some fatal physical condition to overtake the dog, so that they would be spared the anguish of requiring euthanasia for behavioural reasons.

There was evidence from the rest of the dog's behaviour that he saw himself as dominant in the household. Most of the time he did not seek the family's company, but approached them to remind them of meal and walk times and to make the ambiguous social advances already described. When the concept of dominance was explained to Mr. and Mrs. H., they accepted it eagerly. They had not thought of it before, but they now realised that they looked on the dog as an irascible old relative, whose wishes must always be borne in mind and deferred to.

The dog was given a course of megestrol and Mr. and Mrs. H. given instructions outlined above as to how to reduce dominance. When they became more dominant over the dog, they were gradually to start patting him again.

When seen again two weeks later, they reported that Henry had initially seemed confused and bewildered (this is the typical reaction of a dog at the beginning of a dominance reversal regime). He then became more withdrawn, initiating fewer interactions with the owners. There were no aggressive episodes, except one which occurred in a situation which had not previously provoked aggression. While on the higher dose of megestrol, Henry's appetite increased and he started to search the kitchen floor for scraps. While eating one of these scraps, Mr. H. brushed past him and was bitten on the ankle. It seemed that this behaviour was, at least, partly a result of a side-effect of the megestrol and, in fact, did not recur once the drug was withdrawn.

When seen six weeks later, Mr. and Mrs. H. were pleased with the result of treatment. Henry had not snapped again, although he had his 'off days' when he was slow to obey commands. When this happened they went back to a stricter regime of ignoring the dog and rewarding only submissive behaviour. They had clearly understood and used constructively the concepts underlying the treatment methods. The husband had noticed that the wife shouted fiercely at the dog when it did not obey; he pointed out that speaking quietly would be more dominant. They tried this out and found it to be more effective.

TREATMENT METHODS NOT RECOMMENDED

It is often recommended by dog breeders or trainers that the owner of a dominant dog engage in a series of confrontations, hitting it or using other physical means to gain the upper hand. There are several reasons why this course of action is inadvisable:

a.   It is dangerous. Dogs which have already shown dominance aggression are often provoked to attack in such circumstances.

b.   There is a substantial possibility that the dog, not the owner, may win the confrontation. A stranger, such as a veterinary surgeon or dog handler brought in to deal with the problem, stands a greater chance of being successful in confronting the dog as it has not yet established a dominant relationship over him. An owner who is seen as subordinate is more likely to be attacked.

c.   A confrontation of any kind, whether it involves physical violence or shouting at the dog, tends to raise the emotional temperature of the relationship and make it one in which dominance is a 'hot' issue. Although a dog may accept its subordinate relationship temporarily as a result of confrontation, it is more likely to be preoccupied in the long term with winning its dominance back than if an oblique approach is used.

d.   Physical confrontation with the dog carries all the disadvantages of punishment outlined in Chapter 3.11. More specifically, although in this context the dog may cease to show dominance aggression towards the owner, the probability of its showing aggression elsewhere may be increased. An extreme example of this is the brutalising effect of harsh training methods involving a great deal of physical punishment. Dogs subjected to such a regime may be subordinate to their handlers, but unreliable with strangers. Although few owners would be tempted to be so extreme in their methods, it is better to advocate an approach which involves no risk of this kind of effect.

e.   To make a dog afraid is not the same as asserting dominance over it (see Chapter 4.7).

9.3 POSSESSIVE AGGRESSION

The threat in these cases is presented by someone trying to remove something from the dog; most commonly this is food, but some dogs may steal and guard other household items such as underwear, gloves or wallets. This is normally a manifestation of dominance aggression, with the dog showing other signs of dominance within the family. A learned component of the behaviour is usually evident in so far as the dog is rewarded by each incident where it successfully retains possession.

Treatment is as for dominance aggression, as outlined in 9.2: it is directed both in general at altering the dog's dominant position within the family and in particular at changing the possessive behaviour. Where the possessiveness is of objects rather than food, it is often most easily altered by a form of systematic desensitization in which the dog is presented with a hierarchy of increasingly attractive trophies, starting with objects which the dog finds only mildly desirable, perhaps in a location where the dog is less dominant (e.g the garden). The owner should keep a hold on the object at the same time offering it to the dog. When the dog takes it, he should give a specific word of command (e.g. 'leave') and offer an attractive food reward; when the dog relinquishes the object, it gets the food and is praised at the same time. To begin with, the food reward should be clearly more desirable to the dog than the trophy. This gives the owner a chance to teach the 'leave' response, before moving very gradually on to objects which are in more realistic competition with the food. The food reward is gradually phased out, so that the dog is eventually rewarded with praise alone. When food is guarded, rather than objects, the problem is often improved by feeding a less palatable diet, such as a dried complete food. An added advantage of this type of food is that, as a temporary solution to the problem, it need not be fed to the dog in its dish at all; the day's rations are spread throughout the day and hand-fed by the owner as rewards for obedience to commands. Meanwhile, the dog is taught not to guard its dish. One method is to put the dog on a lead which is passed around the table leg in such a way that when the owner is beside the food bowl, he can stop the dog from approaching by pulling on the lead. In this way, the owner controls the dog's access to the food and can make it conditional on the dog sitting on command and showing no aggression (Neville, 1990).

Possessive aggression and pseudopregnancy

Bitches sometimes display possessive aggression as part of a pseudopregnancy. This usually takes the form of guarding small objects (presumably perceived as puppies) often in her bed. The situation is usually best handled by avoiding confrontation but confiscating the objects in the bitch's absence and, if necessary, the bed as well. She should also be distracted with other activities (e.g. play, outings). The aim is to prevent the aggression from being learnt through repetition; it should then subside naturally, along with the other signs of the pseudopregnancy.

9.4 PROTECTIVE AGGRESSION

One manifestation is that the dog defends its territory, which may be the house, the garden or the car, by barking at or attacking outsiders who try to intrude on it. It may object to all intruders or there may be some individuals or types of people (such as men in uniform) whom it particularly dislikes. This attitude may also give rise to the habit of barking at passers-by seen from the window of the car or house, or at the sound of the door-bell or foot-steps approaching. The dog's aggression may be directed towards protecting the owner, rather than its territory. Thus, it may show aggression towards people in the street with whom the owner attempts to converse. If it is particularly attached to one member of the family it may show aggression towards other family members if there are arguments or fights, even in play.

Causes

For about a third of dogs showing protective aggression, this is their only problem and only a quarter also show dominance aggression (Borchelt, 1983), although it seems likely that a greater proportion show other signs of dominance within the family. There must be an inherited component to the behaviour as it is clearly more common in some breeds (e.g. guarding breeds, collies).

In many cases the response seems to have been strengthened through learning. Protective aggression is often shown most violently towards people such as postmen who appear to the dog to be successfully chased away by it. In addition, many owners welcome this kind of aggression when it is, in their eyes, appropriately directed. It is, however, unreasonable to expect a dog to be able to distinguish desirable from undesirable callers by itself. Encouraging a dog's protective instincts and then training it to restrain itself on command is a task only to be undertaken by specialists with specialist dogs (e.g. police dogs).

TREATMENT

A combination of the following methods should be tried:

a.   Where the dog is also showing dominance or dominance aggression towards the family this should be treated.

b. Pre-train the dog in an appropriate alternative response e.g. going to the corner of the hall on command for a reward.

c. Systematically desensitize the dog to the provocative situation, enlisting the help of accomplices. The dog is first of all required to engage in the pre-trained response when a very mild version of the provocative situation occurs. For instance, for dogs which are aggressive towards callers, this might be the sound of foot-steps (pre-arranged) passing the house. At successive stages, the 'visitor' might approach nearer the door, finally ringing the bell and being greeted by the owner.

Over the period of the treatment, the dog should not be exposed to stimuli high on the desensitization hierarchy. For a dog showing aggression towards visitors at the door, this might mean confining it to the back premises except during treatment sessions.

d. An alternative to systematic desensitization is distraction. The barking is interrupted by a startling stimulus (rape alarm, training disks, etc.) which may stop the dog for the few moments necessary for the command for the pre-trained response to be successfully given. Attempts to stop the dog from barking by shouting are normally unsuccessful, as the dog presumably perceives the owner as joining in the barking (Appleby, 1990). Distraction is sometimes successfully provided by a toy (appropriately pre-conditioned: see Chapter 3.10) and kept only for the purpose.

e. Where appropriate, the visitors themselves should give the reward for non-aggressive behaviour.

f. Dogs which cannot be induced to tolerate visitors actually crossing the threshold may have to be shut away until the visitors are settled and sitting down inside: many can then be safely allowed access to the visitors at this point. Alternatively, visitors can sometimes be tolerated if they are first met in the garden (Neville, 1990).

g. More frequent walks and excursions away from home may make some dogs less preoccupied with defending their territory.

h. If the dog's aggression seems to centre around the protection of a family member rather than the protection of territory, the dog's relationship with that person probably needs to be restructured. He may need to increase his dominance over the dog; the relationship may also need to be less exclusive, with other family members or friends becoming more actively involved with the dog.

i. Owners should bear in mind that intervention **before** the aggression occurs is always more likely to be successful.

j. Where there is a risk of the dog actually biting someone, it should be muzzled. In some situations (e.g. around the house) keeping a lead attached to the dog's collar all the time may make it easier to bring it under control.

CASE EXAMPLE 9:2.

Mrs J., a widow in her seventies, sought treatment for Jimmy, a two year-old golden cocker spaniel dog. The problem was that when she took Jimmy in the car with her she could not stop to talk to anyone outside the car without him hurling himself at the other person, barking and growling. She herself had been bitten trying to restrain him. This made transactions such as buying petrol difficult. There was also a problem when she drove into her local village, where she knew most of the inhabitants. Questioning revealed that Jimmy also showed dominance aggression towards her at home. He growled and snapped if she tried to groom him and sometimes when she gave him a command. He slept on her bed, but growled if she inadvertently disturbed him. She commented sadly that she expected this would be her last dog, but she was determined that she would not have him destroyed.

As Mrs. J. lived some distance away, she was seen for only one consultation in person, the rest being conductd by telephone. Jimmy was given megestrol and Mrs. J. instructed how to treat his general dominance, as outlined in 9.2. She was upset by the idea of ignoring him and not allowing him to sleep on her bed, but when it was put to her that this severe regime might eventually be relaxed if the dog's behaviour improved, she agreed to try it. She was delighted to find that Jimmy's aggression towards herself diminished rapidly and she was well motivated to go on to treat the protective aggression. After keeping him at home for a while until she had gained more dominance over him, she started to take him out again to petrol stations. She found that she did not need to enlist the help of an accomplice. It was sufficient to put Jimmy on the floor at the back of the car and tell him to sit before the attendant approached. The dog continued to show aggression towards people who approached the car unexpectedly, but she did not consider this a great problem. The improvement was still maintained at the follow-up, three months after the withdrawal of megestrol.

9.5 FEAR-INDUCED AGGRESSION

The hallmark of this kind of aggression is that it is accompanied by fear, with some of the following characteristics present:

a. The dog's posture is fearful, with its ears and tail down.

b. It does not launch a sustained attack, but typically snaps and withdraws.

c. It occurs when the dog feels unable to escape: either because it is physically restrained, because it is trapped in a confined space or because the perceived threat takes it by surprise.

CAUSES

As with phobias (Chapter 10.1) some cases of fear-induced aggression are explicable in terms of previous unpleasant experiences (e.g. in a veterinary consultation) and in others the cause remains obscure. There seems to be a hereditary component, as this kind of aggression is more common in some breeds e.g. Border collies.

TREATMENT

The treatment of choice is systematic desensitization to the feared situation. Where there is a co-existing dominance (12% show dominance aggression to family members (Borchelt, 1983)) this should be treated.

Veterinary surgeons are often the target of their patients' fear-induced aggression. This may be exacerbated by practitioners who assume that the dog is mounting a dominance challenge and adopt the confrontational approach of shouting at or hitting the dog (see Chapter 4.8). Dogs liable to fear-biting are best approached in a calm, non-threatening way. Fear can be reduced further by spending time with the dog at the beginning of a consultation, interacting with it in a friendly manner.

9.6 NOISE PROVOKED AGGRESSION

In some dogs, aggression seems to be provoked by some high-pitched noises. There seems to be a hereditary factor, as it seems more common in certain breeds (e.g. Rottweilers, terriers). Attacks can be sudden and unpredictable.

CASE EXAMPLE 9.3

In an incident which attracted a good deal of media attention in Scotland, an 11 year old girl, Kellie, was attacked and killed by two Rottweilers. Her friend, Tracy, provided the following details for the fatal accident inquiry.

The girls were on holiday, visiting Tracy's father's hotel and every day they exercised his Rottweilers on leads by the river. A dog and a bitch, they lived in a kennel in the yard by the hotel. Witnesses at the inquiry said the dogs were friendly and generally well behaved; they had been exhibited at shows. On one of these walks, Kellie needed to urinate. Tracy took both the leads and Kellie walked a few yards away. As she crouched down, the dogs lunged towards her and, breaking free from Tracy, ran over to her. At this stage they were friendly and excited; they licked her face. But when Kellie screamed and laughed, they suddenly started to attack her throat. Tracy tried to interpose herself between the dogs and her friend, but they went on attacking. She ran off to fetch her father, but by the time he arrived Kellie was dead. A woman was with him and when she saw the body, she screamed. This provoked the dogs to attack her, but this time the father brought them under control and she was not injured. The dogs were destroyed later the same day by the local veterinary surgeon.

In some noise-provoked attacks, however, there seems to be a learned component. The telephone ringing may cause aggression in some dogs. Often this seems to be only partly because the sound itself is offensive; it is also the signal for the owner's conversation with an unknown stranger. In addition, the owner, in a hurry to answer the telephone, or once engaged in conversation, is not well placed to control the aggression.

TREATMENT

Treatment is similar to other forms of defensive aggression: increasing owner dominance and control, pre-training an alternative response, systematic desensitization. Treatment is more likely to be successful the more precisely the circumstances provoking an attack can be worked out.

CASE EXAMPLE 9:4

Miss P., a lady in her eighties, brought Patsy, a 7 year old Jack Russell terrier bitch, who barked when the telephone rang. More recently, she had started to snap at Miss P.'s ankles as she went to answer it; however, she still barked at the telephone ring alone. There were telephones in both kitchen and sitting room. Sometimes, when Miss P. was in the sitting room and Patsy was shut in the kitchen, she could hear her barking when the telephone rang. She always quietened down once the telephone was picked up, whether she was in the same room as Miss P. or not. As Patsy was also showing general signs of dominance, Miss P. was encouraged to restructure her relationship with her and to pre-train an alternative response of sitting in her basket on command. At the same time, a hierarchy for desensitization was worked out: Miss P. made a tape recording of the telephone and played it to Patsy at gradually increasing volume. This initially provoked barking, but quickly aroused no reaction, however loudly it was played. Ringing the number which causes the exchange to ring back automatically also provoked no reaction, until Miss P. made a move to lift the receiver. It was not clear whether the pattern of behaviour had altered as a result of treatment, or whether the situation had been misconstrued from the start. In any case, Miss P. was now able to use the delay between the telephone ringing and the onset of the aggression to slip Patsy's lead around a table leg and thus bring her under control.

9.7. 'RAGE' SYNDROME

This seems particularly common in whole-colour cocker spaniels, although it can occur in other breeds. The dog attacks suddenly and savagely, without preliminary threats. The owner often reports that during the attack the dog's eyes have a glazed look. Although the owner often experiences the attacks as crazy and completely unprovoked, careful investigation usually reveals that he did something (often involving touching the dog or brushing against it) which it could have interpreted as a dominance challenge or threat of some kind. These dogs usually show other signs of dominance within the family.

TREATMENT

Although it has been reported that primidone produces improvement in 50% of cases (Mugford, 1984) treating the problem by the methods described in this chapter for dominance and other forms of defensive aggression also usually produces some improvement. The prognosis, however, is worse, because of the ferocity of the attacks: a dog with this disorder whose behaviour has improved may still not be tolerable to live with.

CASE EXAMPLE 9:5

A golden cocker spaniel, Danny, owned by Mrs. D., was liable to bite her if she brushed against him, particularly if he was near the refrigerator; he was in the habit of hovering around when she opened its door in the hope of scraps. The dog was much loved and Mrs. D. worked hard at treatment which was directed both towards reducing his general dominance and towards desensitizing him to particular threats.

She achieved significant success and, although the dog sometimes growled at her, he never bit her again. Unfortunately things went wrong at Christmas (often a bad time for dog behaviour problems). The owner's husband was at home (he was a sailor) and her mother-in-law was staying with them. The mother-in-law was helping to wrap presents at the tree and happened to brush against Danny who, up to now, had been merely interested and excited. He turned and bit her. Presents and carpet were covered with blood, mother-in-law was rushed to the doctor in a state of hysteria and Mr. D., who had never liked Danny, was beside himself with rage. Mrs. D. had to bow to majority opinion and Danny was destroyed the same day by the veterinary surgeon.

9.8. MATERNAL AGGRESSION

This form of behaviour, in which a bitch with young puppies threatens people who approach them, may be seen as a variant of dominance aggression, in that her general dominance often also increases at this time. In this case, no attempt should be made to alter the behaviour, which is a normal part of instinctive maternal behaviour.

9.9. AGGRESSION DIRECTED TOWARDS OTHER DOGS

DOGS IN THE SAME HOUSEHOLD

Dogs or bitches may be involved in this form of behaviour. In some cases the dogs may fight at any time, in others only in specific situations, such as when the owner is present, when they are left alone together or when they are in a particular room. The cause is usually some ambiguity or change in the relative dominance status of the two dogs. This may be the result of a change in their relative maturity, as when a puppy is acquired when the other dog is adult, or it may be the result of the owner's behaviour; owners frequently and mistakenly give support to the 'under-dog'. Also, insufficient domination by the owner over either dog may encourage fighting, which is more common among the higher status members of a pack (Chapter 4.10). Sometimes the aggression is the result of extremely complex social situations involving many dogs and family members. It may be almost impossible in these cases to disentangle all the interactions and discover exactly what is going on.

TREATMENT

a.   The owner should consistently reinforce the dominance of the dog which is naturally dominant and the subordinate status of the other. He should do this by giving all rewards, including food and attention, to the dominant dog first. He should particularly take care not to reward any bids for dominance by the subordinate dog.

b.   Castration or administration of megestrol to the subordinate dog or to both may be helpful.

c.   He should attempt to increase his own dominance over both dogs by the means outlined in 9.2.

d.   If possible he should ensure that the dogs are not put into the situations which are most likely to provoke fighting until the dominance hierarchy within the household has been established. The dogs should then be gradually reintroduced to these situations.

DOGS FROM DIFFERENT HOUSEHOLDS

Occasionally a dog shows predatory aggression towards another dog (see 9.1). Normally, however, when a dog attacks another dog, some form of defensive aggression is involved. It may show towards another dog the same range of types of defensive aggression which are shown towards people (9.2 – 9.6). For practical purposes, however, the behaviour can normally be classified as fear induced or dominance aggression.

FEAR-INDUCED AGGRESSION TOWARDS OTHER DOGS

CAUSES

These dogs frequently lack sufficient exposure to other dogs during the socialisation period. As young dogs, they may also have been the victims of an attack by another dog. Their own attacks are a means of dealing with the threat other dogs are perceived as posing. Typically, they are launched on dogs and bitches indiscriminately, without preliminary social interchange between the dogs. However, some of these dogs develop a particular fear of some breeds, perhaps similar to the one which attacked it. Dogs of these and similar breeds may be singled out for attack.

TREATMENT

Treatment should be aimed at gradually re-socialising (i.e. systematically desensitizing) these dogs to other dogs. Ideally, the dog should be introduced to other dogs in a hierarchy, starting with those which are least likely to provoke aggression. In practice, it is often dificult for the owner to find enough other owners who are willing to cooperate in such a treatment regime. Local knowledge is often helpful here; for example, there may be an understanding dog trainer who will allow desensitization to take place in his class. When meeting these other dogs, the patient should be put on an extending lead to keep it under control. A head collar is often useful. If the dog is forced to meet other dogs in a less aggressive posture (i.e. with head to one side and gaze averted), it is less likely to provoke aggression from the other dog. A muzzle may be also be necessary, both actually to prevent biting and to reassure the owners of the other dogs.

DOMINANCE AGGRESSION TOWARDS OTHER DOGS

This is usually, but not always, shown by male dogs towards other male dogs. There is normally some kind of social exchange, involving threats, before the attack, although dogs which are old enemies may not bother with this. The aggression is often worse when the dog is on what it perceives to be its own territory, which may include the local park. Protective aggression may mean that it is also worse when the owner is close by.

TREATMENT

a. The owner should increase his own dominance over the dog. This may reduce the dog's urge to dominate other dogs. It should also enable the owner to exert more control, so that he can more effectively prevent a fight.

b. Inter-male aggression may be improved by castration. In a study by Hopkins (1976), 60% responded favourably. Before undertaking the operation, delmadinone (Tardak, Syntex) should be administered to judge its probable effect.

c. If the situation has reached a crisis or the owner is opposed to castration, megestrol could be used temporarily to reduce the dog's dominance.

d. The dog should be systematically desensitized to possible opponents by the same method as for fear-induced aggression, using a head collar, extending lead and muzzle if necessary.

9.10. GENERAL CONSIDERATIONS

Aggression in dogs can be a worrying problem for the veterinary surgeon because of the danger to others. It often arouses emotion in both owner and veterinary surgeon which can make it difficult for all parties to work out the best course of action. A few owners consciously revel in and encourage their dogs' aggression; others accept that aggression is part of a dog's behavioural repertoire and take measures to keep it under control. Many, however, cannot bear the thought that their beloved pet can be dangerous. Some of these react to an episode of aggression by immediately requesting euthanasia. It might be argued that the veterinary surgeon should grasp any opportunity to destroy an aggressive dog, both to eliminate the danger to others and to remove it from the breeding pool. Certainly there are some situations in which euthanasia is clearly indicated: for example, when young children or the elderly are at risk. In these situations, it may well be best for everyone if the euthanasia is carried out immediately.

However, the veterinary surgeon should take care not to be swept along by the owner's emotions. Firstly, it is important to establish how dangerously aggressive the dog really is. For an inexperienced owner, any manifestation of aggression may raise the spectre of a tragedy such as that described in 9.6. Secondly, the possibility of treatment should be considered and, if appropriate, raised with the owner. Many owners do not realise that treatment is possible or that it produces some improvement in most cases. If they have already made a painful decision in favour of euthanasia, the possibility that it might not be necessary may be hard to absorb. It is pointless trying to treat aggression in a dog whose owner would prefer to have it destroyed, but care should be taken to establish that this really is the owner's preference.

Other owners, faced with their dog's aggression, deal with it by denial. They may insist that their growling dog is friendly or that it would not actually bite; they may describe alarming attacks, or near-attacks, with inappropriate emotion: amusement or indifference. In these cases it is the veterinary surgeon, rather than the client, who feels the worry. However, in these cases, his task is similar to that with the overwrought client: to establish the danger actually posed by the dog's aggression, convey this to the client and consider the options available. Some clients may abandon their denial fairly readily particularly if they have taken it up out of fear that they would be blamed for their dog's behaviour or urged to have it destroyed. If the veterinary surgeon confronts them with the problem, firmly but non-judgementally, they may be relieved. To those who continue to deny the problem, the veterinary surgeon can only make sure that they are aware of his opinion and recommendation.

When weighing up the possible risks and benefits of treating a problem of aggression, it is usually wise to make clear that the owner is solely responsible for the dog's behaviour and must ensure that the dog does no harm, either by avoiding dangerous situations or by using a lead and/or muzzle when exposing it to such situations. If the owner is not prepared to take on that responsibility or the veterinary surgeon considers he is not capable of taking it on, then treatment should not be undertaken.

FURTHER READING

NEVILLE, P. (1991). Do Dogs Need Shrinks? Sidgwick & Jackson, London. Chapter 6: Aggression.

VOITH, V. L. and BORCHELT, P. L. (1982). Diagnosis and treatment of dominance aggression in dogs. In: *Symposium on Animal Behaviour. The Veterinary Clinics of North America.* **12**, 4.

Chapter Ten

**Problems of fearfulness: specific phobias, general nervousness;
problems of excitability: in specific situations, with visitors, in the car,
general excitability; destructiveness in the owner's absence.**

This chapter deals with problems caused by emotional over-reactivity. This can be manifested in the form of fear or nervousness, possibly in the case of dogs of introverted personality, or in the form of excitement in the case of extraverted dogs (see Chapter 5.10). Either form of behaviour can occur as an isolated symptom or, in extreme cases, as a habitual mode of reacting.

10.1. PROBLEMS OF FEARFULNESS: SPECIFIC PHOBIAS

It is not uncommon for a dog of otherwise stable personality to develop an isolated phobia: the survey by O'Farrell, described in Chapter 7.1, found that two out of three dogs are afraid of things like vacuum cleaners or thunder-storms. Whether or not this constitutes a problem depends to a large extent on the owner's circumstances. A fear of the sound of gun-shot may make life very difficult if the dog lives in the country, for example, but may not matter if it lives in the town.

CAUSES

a. **Genetic factors**

   It seems likely that a predisposition to develop certain phobias can be inherited. Fear of loud noises, for example, seems more common in Border collies and Labradors.

b. **Early environment**

   Lack of exposure to a stimulus during the socialisation period can predispose a dog to develop a phobia of that stimulus later. Dogs who hate car journeys were often not taken for car rides as puppies.

c. **Later experiences**

   A phobia of previously neutral stimuli can be acquired by association with a traumatic event.

CASE EXAMPLE 10:1.

Bessie, a bearded collie, was brought to me by Miss B., the daughter of the house, a girl in her late teens. Over the past few months, Bessie had developed a terror of going out for a walk in the streets.

When her lead was produced, she cowered away; when it was put on, she strained and pulled to get back in the house. All outings were a tug-of-war. She was perfectly confident when out in the country or in a park; it was the streets which bothered her. To begin with, no one in the family had the least idea of how it started. Because Bessie was most panic-stricken when taken out by Miss B.'s brother, family suspicions were aroused that he had, perhaps, lost his temper with her on some occasion, but he strenuously denied this. As often happens, it was not until Bessie had improved and everyone had relaxed somewhat that Miss B. remembered the relevant incident. Shortly before the fear had developed, they had taken Bessie to a firework display during the Edinburgh Festival. They had gone to Princes Street, where there were huge crowds. A band played the 1812 Overture, plus cannon, rockets and assorted screeches and bangs. Bessie had been terrified, but at the time none of them had made the connection between that incident and her subsequent fear.

More often, however, there is no obvious single traumatic incident; perhaps a series of sub-traumatic incidents have had a cumulative effect (Chapter 5.2). Fortunately, it is not necessary to be sure about the genesis of a phobia in order to treat it successfully.

d. **Owner attitudes**

Owner anxiety is not correlated with a raised incidence or with severity of phobias in the dog. However, the more anxious the owner, the more troubled they are likely to be by any phobia it might have (Chapter 7.3). An anxious owner may interfere with the dog's recovery from a phobia by being over-solicitous and thus rewarding fearful behaviour. In most cases, however, this is not an important factor.

TREATMENT

Systematic desensitisation is the treatment of choice. When properly carried out, the prognosis for a phobia in a dog of otherwise stable personality is extremely good.

The procedure is as follows:

a. The dog is first of all put into a relaxed frame of mind. This might be achieved by petting it, feeding it tit-bits or by giving it a toy to play with, preferably pre-conditioned as a secondary reinforcer (see Chapter 3.10).

b. The dog is exposed to a version of the phobic stimulus which is so mild that it elicits either no anxiety at all or very mild anxiety which decreases quickly to no anxiety.

c. This stimulus is presented to the dog several times, until it is established beyond doubt that it elicits no anxiety.

d. The procedure is repeated with a stimulus of slightly greater intensity and so on until a stimulus of normal intensity can be tolerated.

Care should be taken to observe the following conditions:

a. Over the period of time when the treatment is being carried out, the dog should not be exposed to a normal version of the phobic stimulus. This may mean making special arrangements or postponing the treatment until an appropriate time (e.g. winter time for a thunder phobia).

b. Treatment should proceed very slowly and gradually. If the dog shows increasing, rather than decreasing, anxiety in the presence of the stimulus, this is a sign that the treatment is proceeding too fast. The remedy is to go back a few stages and proceed at a slower pace.

c. Although it is not essential, long treatment sessions (30 – 40 minutes) are more effective than short ones.

d.   It is not unknown for a relapse to occur after successful treatment, especially after the dog has not been exposed to the phobic stimulus for some time. Regular exposure helps to prevent a relapse but, should a relapse occur, the systematic desensitization should be repeated. Usually this does not take as long as when it was first applied.

Bessie, the bearded collie, was desensitized by first of all not taking her out at all. After a week of this, she was so desperate for an outing that she allowed Miss B. to put her lead on and, eventually, to take her round the block. She refused to go out with any other member of the family, however. The solution was for another family member to accompany Bessie and Miss B. on the walk. Her mother did this and, eventually, Bessie was happy for Mrs. B. to take hold of her lead, with Miss B. walking alongside. Miss B. gradually moved ahead of the pair, until, some days later, she could walk so far ahead that part of the time she was out of sight round the corner. In the end, Bessie would go out with Mrs. B., without seeing Miss B. on the walk at all, as long as Miss B. left the house first. Miss B. could hide round the side of the house and then go back inside once Bessie and Mrs. B. had left. The next step was obviously for Miss B.'s brother to do the same as his mother had done; but when they suggested it, he refused, because he was not going to be seen by the neighbours taking part in this odd procession.

TREATMENTS NOT RECOMMENDED

Owners sometimes report that they have tried to treat their dog's fear by repeatedly exposing it to the feared stimulus. The rationale for this procedure is usually that the dog will thereby discover that his fear is groundless and that no unpleasant consequence follows the feared stimulus. Although this is probably how many fearful reactions are unlearned in the natural course of events, when a fear has reached phobic proportions this procedure is useless. The reason is probably that the experience of extreme fear is itself unpleasant (see Chapter 5.2b).

Although behavioural psychologists working with human patients claim to have used successfully the technique of 'flooding', whereby the patient is exposed to an intense version of the feared stimulus until his autonomic fear responses are exhausted, this technique is not recommended. It is unpleasant for the patient and there is a risk of making the phobia worse. With the safer technique of systematic desensitization available, there seems no reason ever to use 'flooding'.

10.2. PROBLEMS OF FEARFULNESS: GENERAL NERVOUSNESS

The dog shows signs of fearfulness in a wide range of situations. In extreme cases, the dogs whole life may be bedevilled by a mass of phobias; there may be so many and they may be of such routine domestic events (e.g. someone dropping something or entering the room) that the dog is in a constant state of fear.

CAUSES

a.   **Genetic factors**

   A study by Murphree (1976) involving selective breeding (see Chapter 5.10) demonstrated that, in dogs, a predisposition to fearfulness can be inherited.

b.   **Early environment**

   Various factors in the dog's early life can cause excessive emotionality:

   i.   In laboratory rodents **neonatal protein deficiency** can produce emotionality later in life (Hart & Hart, 1985). It seems possible, therefore, that puppies which start life as runts are more likely to develop nervous or excitable personalities.

ii.   It is likely that the **nervousness of the bitch** can affect her puppies in the early weeks, tending to make them more nervous also in later life. Scott & Fuller (1965) found that, on various tests of emotional reactivity, puppies tended to obtain scores more similar to their mothers' than to their fathers'.

iii. An **impoverished physical and social environment** during the socialisation period (3—12 weeks) can give rise to general fearfulness later in life (see Chapter 6.2). A painful condition in puppyhood can have the same effect.

c.   **Later experiences**

As with human beings, adverse experiences later in life can permanently affect personality, but they have to be of an extreme nature (e.g. concentration camps in the case of human beings) to produce as profound an effect as early experience. Although dogs can be made generally nervous and fearful by systematically terrorising them, this is rare; a dog of stable personality which is frightened in adult life is more likely to develop an isolated phobic symptom.

d.   **Owner attitudes**

Although an owner's attitudes rarely cause an anxiety state in a dog, they may help to maintain it. When a dog's nervousness is extreme, the owners may be at their wits' end. They may be both intensely irritated by the dog's behaviour and, at the same time, have a guilty feeling that they are somehow responsible for it. This may lead to inconsistent behaviour towards the dog which increases its level of stress. Phobic behaviour may be rewarded with attention and normal behaviour ignored.

TREATMENT

As far as possible, an environment should be temporarily arranged which causes minimal upset to the dog. This may mean not taking it out, muffling bells or making special arrangements when visitors call. The dog's nervous reactions are then treated as separate phobic symptoms by systematic desensitization (see 10.2). In extreme cases, desensitization may not be feasible or it may be ineffective; as soon as one phobia improves, another may appear. Many of these cases improve, however, if their overall stress levels are reduced. Towards this end, and for the sake of the whole family, it may be best to help the owners to resign themselves to having a dog with a disability. They should not make strenuous efforts to cure it, but should work out a *modus vivendi* which is tolerable for all concerned. Thus, they should not force the dog unnecessarily into situations which cause it suffering (e.g. going for walks) but on the other hand they should not disrupt their own routine too much for the dog's sake. The dog's anxious behaviour should be ignored and normal behaviour rewarded.

10.3. PROBLEMS OF EXCITABILITY: IN SPECIFIC SITUATIONS

Many dogs become excited in specific situations, such as in the car, or when visitors arrive. The dog may express his state of high arousal by barking or by dashing to an fro. Or he may perform a displacement activity, such as sexual mounting, digging, tail chasing or chewing (see Chapter 5.4 f).

CAUSES

a.   **Specific Stimuli**

Certain kinds of stimulus such as high pitched noises (which also provoke aggression in some dogs [Chapter 9.6]) are more likely than others to provoke excitement. Other stimuli are more likely to provoke certain displacement activities: for example, in some dogs, shadows can trigger stereotypic chasing, pouncing or digging.

b. **Learning**

A stimulus may provoke excitement because the dog learns, by classical conditioning, to associate it with something interesting or desirable. Thus, the dog may become excited when its dish or lead are produced, as they are usually associated with food or an outing. Instrumental learning may also take place, with the desirable events rewarding the preceding excitement. This latter process is often facilitated by the understandable tendency of the owner to deliver the reward more quickly the greater the excitement. Ineffectual reprimands may constitute a further reward for the behaviour.

c. **Conflict/frustration**

There is often an element of conflict, frustration or uncertainty in a stimulus which produces over-excitement. For example, when the owner picks up the dish or lead, the dog often has to wait for the food to arrive or the door to be opened. Occasionally, the excitement may be produced by family rows or upsets; one owner reported her Jack Russell terrier chewed the carpet when she got cross with her son. Presumably these dogs are in conflict as to what part they should play in the rows. Dogs whose loyalties are less divided may attack the less preferred family member.

TREATMENT

An appropriate combination of the following methods should be tried:

a. **Removal of the exciting stimulus**

In a few cases, this is enough to solve the problem. For example, the destructive chewing of the Jack Russell terrier, triggered by family rows, was reduced to manageable proportions when the mother adopted the policy of shutting the dog in another room before starting to tackle her son about some misdemeanour. This will be only temporarily effective if the stimulus is not intrinsically exciting, but exciting as a result of a learned association with an intrinsically exciting experience. For example, a dog which becomes excited before walks may be temporarily calmed by altering the pre-walk routine: leaving by another door, putting the lead on outside, etc. However, the excitement will return as the dog learns to associate these new stimuli with the prospective walk. In these cases, removing the triggering stimulus should be a prelude to:

b. **Systematic desensitization** (see Chapter 8.8)

CASE EXAMPLE 10:2.

Mac was a German shepherd police dog. He was very good at his job and he and his handler, P.C. M., competed regularly in police dog trials. The problem arose when Mac was in the back of the police van, cruising around between assignments. The backs of these vans were fitted with wire-mesh cages and as soon as Mac was put into one, he would start to whine and bark. When the van started, Mac would take up a stereotypic posture with his nose jammed into the top front corner of the cage, his ears back and a glazed look in his eyes. He progressed from whining, through barking on a high-pitched note, to finally trembling and salivating profusely. P.C. M. was clearly very fond of his dog and was distressed to see him in this state. He said that in all other situations Mac behaved perfectly, even when he travelled in the back of the family car.

The police force had taken Mac over as a puppy from owners who had not been able to cope with him. He had been rather too excitable initially, but P.C. M.'s training had soon calmed him down, for the most part. He had always been restless in the van, however, and lately this had got much worse. P.C. M. had tried shouting at Mac; he had tried squirting water at him; he had tried ignoring him: nothing seemed to make any difference.

There seemed to be several reasons why Mac should be over-excited when he was in the van. He was often agitated when he went there: for example, if hooligans at a soccer match taunted him, he would be put into his kennel for a bit, in case matters got out of hand. Also, when Mac left the van, it was usually either to have a run in the park or to do the work he enjoyed so much. Therefore, for much of his time in the van, he was in a high state of anticipation. Added to this, there was the stress produced by confinement. It also seemed possible that the dog was upset at being separated from P.C. M. To explore this latter possibility, P.C. M. tried driving the police van with Mac sitting in the front passenger seat; it turned out that he was quite calm when he sat there.

The problem was then treated by systematic desensitization, using a hierarchy of increasing degrees of separation from P.C. M. The cage was taken out of the back of the van and for a few days Mac rode around in the back of the van with his head on his handler's shoulders. Then he spontaneously gave that up and settled down in a more comfortable position on the floor. P.C. M. then put up a wire-mesh barrier between the front seats and the back of the van; this separated Mac from his handler but left him the freedom of all the back of the van. He tolerated this perfectly well.

But P.C. M. was in a hurry to make his arrangements seem more orthodox, before they attracted the adverse attention of his superiors. He made the mistake of hurrying the systematic desensitization along too fast. He put up another wire-mesh barrier, at right angles to the first: this made a sort of cage. When he came for his next appointment, this had been in place for two days. Mac had clearly not liked it and had whined, though not as badly as before. P.C. M. knew he had been rushing things; he agreed to dispense with the second barrier altogether for a while and then to introduce it in gradual stages: perhaps starting with one which was only a foot high and then gradually increasing its height.

c.   **Rearrangement of rewards**

The rewards maintaining the behaviour are made contingent on calm behaviour. Excitable behaviour is not rewarded. Thus, if the dog becomes excited when the lead is produced, the lead is immediately replaced. It is only produced again when the dog is calm. The dog often learns more quickly if this procedure is accompanied by:

d.   **Distraction and response substitution** (see Chapter 8.8).

CASE EXAMPLE 10:3.

Miss L. was a school teacher who lived with her elderly mother. When she rang me to make an appointment she said that it was 'on behalf of a little black poodle'. But the poodle, Leo, did not seem particularly eager to get help. He seemed to be enjoying himself in an over-enthusiastic sort of way, running round the consulting room, jumping on everyone's knee, all the time giving out a continuous stream of high-pitched yaps so loud and piercing that it was impossible to converse. Miss L. was nearly in tears. When the dog was eventually put in another room, Miss L. was able to say that at home Leo was quiet and well behaved. It was only in a strange house that he would behave in this way. She told me that when Leo became very excitable he would grab her arm or her hostess's arm with his front paws and sexually mount it; this was clearly a displacement activity.

It was explained to Miss L. that Leo's over-excitement was rewarded by everyone's attention. When he was brought back into the room, he was to be ignored completely by everyone. He was frantic for the first five minutes, yelping and jumping. He then started to calm down and eventually sat at Miss L.'s feet. Following instructions, at this point she patted him and told him he was a good dog.

COMMON PROBLEMS OF EXCITABILITY

10.4. EXCITEMENT WITH VISITORS

The dog may greet visitors with uncontrollable exuberance, barking, jumping up and pawing for attention. It may react in a more ambivalent way, barking from a distance or racing about the house, without coming into direct contact with the visitor.

CAUSES

Visitors are common focus of excitable behaviour, probably because dogs are such social animals that a new person is naturally of great interest and is a potential source of rewarding attention. The dog may be frustrated by having to wait for this attention: the louder it barks, the sooner it is liable to be greeted. In addition, there is usually no set ritual of greeting, known to both parties, as there is for a dog and family members; this adds to the uncertainty. At the same time, many dogs are thrown into a state of conflict as to whether the visitor should be construed as a pack member to be greeted or an intruder to be warned off.

TREATMENT

The problem may be treated along the same lines as protective aggression towards visitors (Chapter 9.4) i.e. by response substitution. The response could be some action, such as sitting in a particular place in the hall, which visitors can reward with their attention. Visitors should be instructed not to pay attention to the dog until it is sitting calmly in the proper place. Alternatively, the response could be a self-rewarding one, such as playing with a favourite toy, onto which the dog can displace his excitement. The toy should be kept by the door and used only for this purpose. To begin with, the dog should be shut away when visitors arrive who are too exciting or cannot be trusted to ignore an excited dog.

10.5. EXCITEMENT IN THE CAR

When in a car, the dog is restless, even to the point of becoming a safety hazard. It may bark, pant or salivate. It may even chew the seat-belts or try to dig up the car seats. This behaviour may start immediately the dog gets into a car, when it is in the car and sees the owner approaching or when the car starts moving. It may happen only in certain cars, with certain people or on certain journeys. It is important to find out the details of the stimuli which trigger the behaviour in each individual case, because the treatment plan depends on them.

Sometimes the owners have to carry out some experiments (e.g. with different drivers or different journeys) before the stimuli can be exactly specified.

Protective aggression (see Chapter 9.4) in the car can be sometimes confused with excitement. In these cases the dog barks at people or other dogs, especially if they approach the car. The barking is accompanied by growling or threatening behaviour; sometimes the owner is snapped at if he tries to control the dog.

CAUSES

a. The motion of a car or the noise of the engine seem to be stimuli which can cause agitation in dogs, unless they become accustomed to them from an early age. Dogs which develop problem behaviour in cars are somtimes found to have been introduced to them after the socialisation period (see Chapter 6.2).

b. Excitement can also be produced by the frustrating nature of cars: interesting but inaccessible things are visible out of the windows.

c. There is often both an element of classical conditioning and instrumental learning in the excitement.

    i. Classical conditioning may occur when the dog associates getting into the car, or the car starting, with the imminent appearance of interesting sights out of the window and perhaps with a walk at the end of the journey.

ii.   The excitable behaviour can also be instrumentally learned. As the car continues on its journey, the dog's barking or jumping about is often rewarded by interesting and new sights, or by the sight of the starting place of a walk; it seems to the dog as if its restlessness had brought about this desirable result. The owner's attempts to distract the dog, soothe it or grab hold of it while driving the car often act as additional rewards.

TREATMENT

a. **Systematic desensitization and response substitution**

The dog is pre-trained to sit on command in the stationary car, if this does not excite it. During a training session it is told to sit in the car and the owner proceeds gradually through a hierarchy of stimuli, the dog being rewarded as long as it remains calm. A typical hierarchy might consist of putting the key in the ignition without turning it, turning on the engine and immediately turning it off again, leaving the engine running for longer periods, eventually driving the car very short distances. The success of this procedure depends on having accurately determined the relevant stimuli beforehand. During the period of the treatment, the dog should not be taken on real car trips.

b. **Rearrangements of rewards**

Calm behaviour should be rewarded rather than excitement. The owner should ignore the dog when it is excited, unless he can intervene effectively. The reward of the car proceeding on its journey can be removed by stopping the car as soon as the dog gets excited and only restarting when the dog is calm.

c. **Distraction and response substitution**

The dog's excitement is interrupted by a startling sound (e.g. training disks, rape alarm) and the command for the pre-trained response of sitting is given.

d. Caging the dog or restraining it by means of a harness so that it cannot see out of the car window may be helpful.

e. In some cases being separated from the owner may be a factor in the excitement. Allowing the dog in the front seat may be helpful but it may be necessary, in the interests of safety, to restrain it with a harness.

10.6. GENERAL EXCITABILITY

These dogs are constantly restless and overactive. They may react with uncontrollable excitement to a whole range of stimuli. They engage in a displacement activity or stereotypy, or a variety of such activities, throughout the day. Typically, owners report that no amount of exercise seems to tire the dog out and that it can eat any amount of food without getting fat.

When the dog's activities are bizarre and repetitive, a diagnosis of epilepsy may seem tempting. However, it is usually easy to demonstrate that the movements of the dog are voluntary and purposive, rather than involuntary (for example, it may avoid obstacles or attempt to evade or escape from a restraining hand) and the diagnosis can be excluded.

CAUSES

a. **The same genetic, constitutional and early environmental** factors can contribute to excitability as to fearfulness (see 10.2).

b.   **Learning.** There is a natural tendency for owners to pay more attention to the dog when it is behaving in an excitable or peculiar way than when it is calm. Some owners will speak pleasantly to the dog in an attempt to calm or distract it; others will reprimand the dog. In either case, the dog is being rewarded by the owner's attention.

c.   **Conflict and owner attitudes.** It has been found (Chapter 7.4) that owner neurosis is correlated with various forms of excitable behaviour in the dog. It was argued that this is probably because neurotic owners are more likely to give their dogs contradictory messages, thus producing a state of conflict and therefore a state of heightened arousal. The same effect can probably be produced by busy households with many family members, particularly children. If a consistent regime for the dog has not been agreed on, it can become confused.

TREATMENT

a.   ### Individual symptoms

It is worth trying to treat individual symptoms in the way described in 10.3. If the behaviour only occurs when the owner is present, then it can be inferred that the owner is rewarding it in some way. He should be instructed to ignore the dog whenever the behaviour starts, to the extent of leaving the room if necessary. He should reward the dog when it behaves normally. If the behaviour continues when the owner is absent (e.g. the dog can be seen chasing its tail in the garden or heard doing it at night), then it is almost certainly self-rewarding. In these cases, when the owner is present, he should intervene at the onset of the behaviour, with distraction and response substitution.

b.   ### Lowering stress levels

Most of these dogs and their owners are caught up in a vicious circle. The owner, worried and perhaps also irritated by his dog's behaviour, pays the dog attention when it engages in the behaviour, thus rewarding it. Moreover, the owner, in his anxiety, often alternately and inconsistently shows solicitude and anger towards the dog, thus putting it into a state of conflict and uncertainty and further raising its level of stress. In these cases, pointing out to the owner what is happening and reassuring him that the dog is not physically ill and that its behaviour is capable of change is often enough to break the vicious circle.

In many cases, however, the owner's anxiety is also fuelled by stresses other than the dog's behaviour, such as a physical or mental illness, bereavement, family conflict, etc. It is often clear that the dog is being used as a 'lightning conductor' for some of the unmanageable emotion (see Chapter 7.3). However, these dogs are failing in this role. To extend the metaphor, they are channelling the lightning back into the house with the voltage increased.

It may seem intrusive and potentially counter-productive to point out these processes to a client. However, there are many who can make use of such an insight, especially if it is put to them tactfully and non-judgementally, perhaps in the form of a hypothesis. Obviously, they cannot solve their personal and family problems to order, but they can take steps to protect the dog from stress by, for example:

i.   Making its routine as stable as possible.

ii.   Reaching a policy decision in the family as to what the dog is and is not allowed to do.

iii.   Trying not to make the dog the focus of extremes of emotion. The owner should not punish the dog or shout at it. He should try not to use it excessively as a source of comfort, either.

c. **Drug treatment**

Where a stereotypy is resistant to behavioural treatment, it is worth trying a long-acting morphine antagonist, such as Naltrexone (Nalorex, Du Pont). Morphine antagonists have been shown to reduce significantly stereotypic grooming in dogs (Dodman *et al*, 1988) and other stereotypies in pigs and horses. This class of drugs presumably works by reducing the self-rewarding effect of the stereotypy, which can be viewed as a kind of addiction. The drug can, therefore, create a window of opportunity to teach the dog acceptable, non-stereotypic forms of activity. Its administration is unlikely to result in long-term success unless behavioural methods, such as response substitution are employed simultaneously and the stress causing the stereotypy reduced.

d. **Diet**

It is worth experimenting with a low-protein lamb and rice diet (see Chapter 8.7).

CASE EXAMPLE 10:4.

Mrs. I. and her teenage son, Ian, came for help with their German shepherd dog Ivan. Mrs. I. looked pale and dishevelled. She talked non-stop in an agitated and incoherent way. Ian looked embarassed. Ivan's trouble had started a few months before, when he became very restless. This restlessness now took a different, annoying form at various times of the day. In the morning, when members of the family prepared to leave for work or school, he circled round and round them. When he and Mrs. I. were left alone togther, he tried to follow her everywhere around the house, even into the lavatory. When he was with her, he would dash to and fro, twining around her legs. If she shouted at him, he would sit quietly for a moment and then start again. If she left the house, he would become really frantic and she usually found some damage done when she returned. The Venetian blinds had been destroyed (presumably in his attempts to look for her out of the window). When everyone was at home in the evening, Ivan behaved reasonably enough, but when they started to go to bed, he became restless again. He would dash from one bedroom to another. Often he would jump on and off Ian's bed and try to squeeze between Ian and the bedhead, which, given his size, was impossible.

Mrs. I. said the behaviour had got worse since an incident involving a chip pan which caught fire. The fire brigade had been called, several firemen had rushed in and drenched the kitchen in water. She thought that had quite upset him. There was something about the detached way in which she described her part in the fire, as if she did this kind of thing all the time, which raised questions as to whether she was completely well.

Further probing revealed that she had recently had a 'breakdown' and had been off work. She had panic attacks, in which she sweated, her heart raced and she thought she was going to die. These often happened in the middle of the night and she would telephone her G.P., who would have to come and talk her down. He would tell her that she was not having a heart attack yet. She said she thought Ivan probably felt the same kind of panic when he was in one of his states.

It also emerged that Ivan was really Ian's dog. They had got him when he was a year old from a family who had neglected him, keeping him tied up all day. Ian, who was fifteen at the time, had been in trouble with the police and was truanting from school; Ivan had been intended as a sort of therapy for Ian. This therapy had been outstandingly successful — Ian had been devoted to Ivan and his behaviour had improved dramatically. But, Mrs. I. complained, lately Ian had been neglecting Ivan. He was out with his friends in the evenings and did not pay Ivan any attention, let alone take him out for walks. At this point, Ian protested that he did attend to Ivan when he was at home and that he took him for long walks at weekends.

In this first consultation, an attempt was made to persuade Mrs. I. that whatever had happened to Ivan in the past, he was perfectly well cared for now and not neglected; he was quite capable of adapting to the reduced amount of attention from Ian that he was now receiving. It was a mistake for Mrs. I. to suppose that he was feeling panicky like her; he had simply got into a set of bad habits which he would have to unlearn. The I's were also advised to make sure that Ivan's over-activity was never rewarded by their attention. They were to make a fuss of him only when he was calm. Mrs. I. was to be especially careful to ignore him before she went out (see 10.7: Destructiveness in the owner's absence). In order to treat the night time problem, the I's were to change some aspects of their bedtime routine: they were to leave a light on in the hall and Ian was to change bedrooms with his brother. The aim of these changes was to mislead Ivan, if only temporarily, and so allow an opportunity for more calm behaviour, which could be rewarded. As far as possible, the pacing and bed-jumping were to be ignored.

Mrs. I. came on her own for the next appointment. She seemed calmer and said that Ivan was better. She was vague about the details of his improvement, but it was established that there had been no more episodes of destruction. She seemed more interested in talking about her group therapy sessions at the local hospital. She said these had made her panic attacks easier to cope with.

The final contact with the family was with Ian on his own. He confirmed that Ivan was improving, but he wanted to expand on an aspect of the situation which so far had only been touched on. He said that his mother nagged him constantly about his neglect of Ivan. He had a girl friend now and was planning to move into a flat with her: Ivan would come too. It was pointed out to him that Mrs. I. was indirectly expressing her objections to his increasing independence and to his having a girl friend, by making him feel guilty about Ivan. He was again assured that he had no need to feel guilty and Ivan's best interests were served by ignoring Mrs. I's criticisms: the less Ivan were used as a pawn in family emotional games, the calmer he would become.

10.7. DESTRUCTIVENESS IN THE OWNER'S ABSENCE

Logically, this should be classified as excitement in a specific situation. However, it often shows many of the features of general over-excitement. It is also the commonest major behaviour problem after aggression.

Typically, when left alone in the house the dog engages in frantic chewing or digging behaviour which may be directed against the door, carpet, furniture or objects of the house. The dog may also urinate or defaecate. It may also howl or bark; many dogs do only this, without accompanying destructive behaviour. This can constitute a problem if the noise disturbs neighbours.

The behaviour sometimes occurs when the owners are in the house, but have shut the dog away from them overnight. It can also occur in cars, although dogs which are destructive in cars do not necessarily show the behaviour in the house and vice versa. The dog may not be destructive every time it is left alone. A common pattern is that it behaves normally during separations which occur routinely (such as when the owner goes to work) but may be destructive during unexpected separations.

CAUSES AND TREATMENT

By far the commonest cause of this behaviour is the dog's agitation at being left alone. As they are pack animals, dogs instinctively become uneasy if separated from the rest of the pack, particularly the leader. The chewing and digging are displacement activities produced by the increase in anxiety level, which can also result in uncontrolled urination and defaecation. In some situations (e.g. if the dog scratches at the door), some of the behaviour can also be seen as an attempt to follow the rest of the pack; the howling and barking as attempts to attract its attention.

Typically, the dogs which react adversely to separation are those which are suddenly faced with relatively long periods of solitude, having previously always had company. Problems often arise after a holiday or after radical changes in the owner's life-style.

When the owner is at home, these dogs usually follow him around everywhere. A traumatic event occurring when the dog is left alone can precipitate anxiety. It is also more common in dogs from rescue organisations (McCrave & Voith, 1986). Presumably their history of traumatic separations has made them more prone to over-attachment to a permanent owner.

A dog whose destructive behaviour is a reaction to separation is usually affected by the sight of the owner preparing to go out. It usually becomes agitated although it may become aggressive to the owner or withdrawn and dejected. The destruction usually occurs just after the owner has left, perhaps preceded by some other agitated activity, such as barking or wandering around. Many owners already have evidence as to when the behaviour occurs, usually as a result of having gone back to collect something soon after they have left the house. If not, it is helpful if they can find this out, either by returning stealthily to the house or by leaving a tape recorder running. In addition, dogs which suffer from separation anxiety normally greet their owners on their return with enormous excitement, although some may slink away if they have learned to expect punishment.

TREATMENT

Treatment should consist of an appropriate combination of the following methods:

a.   The relationship between dog and owner should be restructured to make them less mutually dependent. The owner should be encouraged to pay as little attention to the dog as possible until the problem is under control. They should be particularly careful not to respond to the dog's demands for attention or for anything else.

b.   The dog may be systematically desensitized to the owner's departure. The first stage is often to desensitize the dog to being alone in a room. The dog is trained to sit in his bed (see e. below) on command. It is then rewarded for staying there while the owner progressively withdraws further from the dog, going out of sight for increasing lengths of time. The reward should always be given to the dog sitting in his bed or cage. Approaching the owner should not be rewarded. The dog should then be desensitized to departures from the house in the same way. The owner begins by rewarding the dog for sitting calmly during the normal pre-departure routine (picking up keys, handbag etc.). The owner should then leave and return immediately; the length of absence should then be gradually extended, always rewarding only calm behaviour on return. If at any point the dog's agitation starts to increase, it is a sign that the desensitization is proceeding too quickly. Over the period that the treatment is being carried out, the dog should not be subjected to real separations which it cannot tolerate. This may mean making dog-sitting arrangements or carrying out the treatment during a holiday.

c.   If the triggering stimuli (i.e. the events which the dog had learnt to associate with departure) are altered, its agitation at the actual departure may be lessened, at least temporarily. Thus, the owner might leave by a different door, having left his coat in the car, or he might carry something the dog has learnt to associate with immediate return e.g. a milk bottle. Giving the dog something to chew while it is alone may be helpful. This should be given before the pre-departure routine which agitates the dog. Rawhide chews may not last long enough to be practical. A nylon chew is better from this point of view; its attractiveness may be enhanced by boring small holes in it and filling them with cheese. The chew should be removed on the owner's return to maintain its novelty value.

d.   Confining the dog in a small space or cage is likely to increase its agitation if done abruptly. If a cage is introduced slowly as part of a systematic desensitization programme (see b.) it can give a dog a feeling of security. The cage should be made as inviting as possible, by putting the dog's familiar blanket, toys, etc. in it.

e.   The owner should ignore the dog for 15 – 20 minutes before departure and on return. This helps to lessen the contrast between the owner's presence and his absence.

f.   Getting another dog is a solution which owners often contemplate, but it is a risk. The result may be two destructive dogs. It is most likely to be successful with dogs which have a history of close bonding with other dogs and especially in dogs whose destructiveness has been precipitated by the death of another dog in the household.

g.   Lowering stress levels is often important in these cases. An owner's insight into the process which led him to become over-involved with the dog may make disengagement easier. The extent of damage done by some of these dogs puts the owner/dog relationship under severe strain and propels it into a vicious circle of increased anger on the owner's part leading to increased stress and, therefore, increased destructiveness by the dog. If the owner can be persuaded not to show anger towards the dog the consequent lowering of the dog's level of stress may, on its own, bring about some improvement in behaviour.

Punishment or even speaking crossly to the dog should be avoided. The dog can make no sense of the owner's displeasure when it occurs hours after the episode of destruction; it can only make it more agitated. Owners sometimes refuse to accept this, saying that when the dog has been destructive it looks 'guilty' on the owner's return. In fact the 'guilt' is fear of punishment, which the dog has learnt to associate with the presence of debris. This is different from associating punishment with the act of creating the debris.

ADDITIONAL FACTORS

There may be other factors involved in some instances of destructive behaviour. These factors may occasionally operate on their own, but there is usually some degree of separation anxiety present.

a.   **Boredom seems to encourage some destructive behaviour**
When they have been left alone for a period, some dogs' need for activity and stimulation increases to the point at which they engage in displacement behaviour. Boredom is likely to be a causative factor if the destruction does not take place immediately after the owner has left but after the dog has rested for a while. Young active dogs are more likely to engage in this type of destruction, as are dogs which are left for longer periods than a dog would normally sleep during the day i.e. more than 3 or 4 hours. The only solution in this type of situation is for the owner to make alternative arrangements for the dog during his absence or find another home where the owners would not be absent for such long periods.

b.   **Some episodes of destruction seem to be triggered by an event occurring during the owner's absence**
This may be something which triggers territorial aggression, such as a caller ringing the bell or putting something through the letter box. It may be a phobic stimulus such as thunder. If these stimuli are relevant, the dog usually reacts to them when the owner is present, though not always with the same vigour.

The best hope of modifying destructive reactions to such stimuli is systematic desensitization. In most cases, it may be possible to confine the dog to a part of the house where it does not hear these sounds so clearly.

CASE EXAMPLE 10:5

Mrs. T., a nurse in her twenties, came for advice about her Doberman, Tommy. When she was out at work, he would get hold of any loose objects lying around (for example, books, tapes or cushions) and reduce them to shreds. She knew he did it soon after she left, because on one or two occasions she had come back unexpectedly for something she had forgotten. He always became very agitated before she left and was extremely excited when she returned. Mr. T. was a soldier, who had been away for the last two months on a training course, only coming home for odd weekends. He was fond of Tommy, but was quickly losing patience. He said that if this problem was not sorted out by the time his course was over, Tommy would have to go. Mrs. T. was deeply attached to Tommy and felt that to part with him would be the end of the world. She talked lovingly about all his little ways and on the telephone would announce herself as 'Tommy's mummy', which was confusing.

It was explained to Mrs. T. that although it was natural that she depend on Tommy while her husband was away, the emotional closeness that had sprung up between them was making him miss her a great deal when she was out. The remedy was to pay him much less attention: in fact, when Mr. T. was at home, he should take over Tommy's care and Mrs. T. should ignore Tommy completely. Although the thought of doing this distressed her, she saw the sense of it. She was also very keen not to lose Tommy. When she came again, it was with her husband who was on leave; they reported that Tommy was much calmer and that there had been no further episodes of destruction.

FURTHER READING

MUGFORD, R. (1984). Car crazy: dog travel in cars. Pedigree Digest 11.2

VOITH, V. L. and BORCHELT, P. L. (1985). Separation anxiety in dogs. The Compendium on Continuing Education for the Practising Veterinarian. 7,1. 42-52.

VOITH, V. L. and BORCHELT, P. L. (1985). Fears and phobias in companion animals. The Compendium on Continuing Education for the Practising Veterinarian. 7,3. 209-218.

MISCELLANEOUS PROBLEMS

Chapter Eleven

Coprophagia and pica; anorexia; obesity; inappropriate urination and defaecation; inappropriate sexual mounting; uncontrollable behaviour on walks.

EATING PROBLEMS

11.1. COPROPHAGIA AND PICA

It is common for dogs to eat a wider range of substances than their owners find acceptable. In the absence of dietary deficiency, there are various possible reasons for this:

a. **Many dogs seem to have an instinctive preference for food which is decaying.** This leads them to eat rotting carcases, faeces and the contents of dust-bins. In addition, part of a dam's instinctive behavioural repertoire is eating her puppies' stools. Coprophagia and carrion eating are, therefore, normal behaviour, but many owners find them repellent and they do expose the dog to extra risk of infection and parasites. There are various ways of attempting to modify the behaviour:

   i.   Deny the dog access to the tempting substances for some weeks. Dogs which eat their own faeces must be supervised whenever they defaecate: immediately they have finished, they must be distracted and another response substituted (e.g. coming indoors for a tit-bit). Similarly, a dog which eats the faeces of other animals or carrion should be closely supervised on walks and distraction and response substitution used whenever it approaches or starts looking for these items. It may be necessary to use an extending lead and/or muzzle. Once a new routine of activities has been established at the relevant times, the owner may be able gradually to withdraw his supervision.

   ii. The dog's appetite may be reduced by feeding lesser amounts more often and by adding fibre to the diet to promote a feeling of fullness.

   iii. Interruption/aversion (e.g. rape alarm, training disks) can be applied just before the dog picks up the stool. If the owner is prepared to try it, the stool may be booby trapped (e.g. with cap bangers).

   iv. Where the dog eats its own stool this may be made less palatable by modifying the diet by

      a. feeding a diet high in fibre and protein, low in carbohydrate.

b. giving an iron supplement.

　　c. adding vegetable oil, increased over a week to 15ml/4.5 kg body weight (McKeown *et al,* 1988).

b.　A dog's mouth is the organ by means of which it explores and takes possession of objects as well as eating them. Sometimes the functions become confused so that **the dog ends up by partially ingesting something which it had originally intended only to investigate or remove.** This can become a problem when the objects are dangerous to the dog (e.g. stones) or precious to the owner. The following treatment methods may be tried:

　　i.　If there is possessive aggression involved (i.e. the dog growls or threatens when the owner tries to take the object away) this should be treated (see Chapter 9.3).

　　ii.　The owner's reaction, which may include an enjoyable chase, may be rewarding. Where this seems to be the case, the owner should be instructed, where feasible, to ignore the dog when he sees it with something already in its mouth: the optimum time for intervention — as the dog approaches the object — having already passed.

　　iii.　When the owner sees the dog approaching the object he should intervene with distraction and response substitution. To make this possible, increased supervision of the dog is often necessary.

11.2. ANOREXIA

Occasionally, dogs may become reluctant to eat from other than physical causes: this most commonly happens following a change of environment or loss of a person or animal to which the dog is attached. Thus, a dog may not eat when it is put in boarding kennels, goes to a new home, or if a human or animal member of the family dies or goes away. This behaviour may appear on its own or may be part of a clinical picture which includes withdrawn or listless behaviour and which seems comparable with mourning or depressive reactions in human beings.

In most cases, given time and patience, appetite returns; it may be necessary to tempt the dog with tasty foods and hand-feed it. In some cases, however, the anorexia persists so long as to give cause for concern. Where no physical problem can be discovered, it often emerges that the owners are maintaining the food refusal by their own behaviour. They may be so worried that they continually pester the dog with food or try to force it to eat, so making the whole feeding situation unpleasant. If this appears to be happening, the owners should be instructed to offer appetising food at set times, say twice daily, leave the dog to investigate it on its own and remove it after 5—10 minutes. It may prove helpful if the dog can stay for a few days in another household which is not associated with unpleasant feeding experiences and whose members are not so emotionally involved in the problem.

11.3. OBESITY

It may seem odd to include in a book on dog behaviour problems a problem which is so clearly due to the owner's behaviour. However, as has been argued in earlier chapters, most dog behaviour problems are, to some extent, a product of interaction between dog and owner. The same applies to over-eating. The difference between this condition and other behaviour problems is that the action required of the owner is simply stated: to give the dog less food. However, persuading an owner to do this can be as difficult a task of modifying attitudes as in any other behavioural problem.

An owner may overfeed her dog for various reasons:

a.　**She may imagine that her dog's need for food is the same as hers:** that it only feels satisfied if it has breakfast, lunch, dinner and tea and feels deprived if it is fed less often. It may be necessary to explain to her that a dog's digestive system is designed to receive enormous amounts of food as long as they are available, in the expectation of many days fasting. It is normal and healthy for a dog to be keen to eat most of the time, but this eagerness does not mean it is experiencing an actively unpleasant sensation of 'hunger'. Some owners find this a difficult concept to grasp and others are too emotionally involved with their dogs to be willing to grasp it.

b.   **It gives many owners great satisfaction to give their dogs pleasure by feeding them.** When this mutually gratifying interaction is replaced by a dog which looks reproachful or whines and pesters for more, it is often more than the owner can bear. In addition, feeding the dog tit-bits is often built into the social fabric of the day (e.g. 'When I have coffee and a biscuit, he always gets a bit'). It has been observed (Leigh, 1966) that obese dogs are likely to have obese owners but the issue is probably more complex than that. Everyone feels anxious if their sources of security are threatened; for some people this feeling of security is closely bound up with food and eating. These people are not necessarily obese themselves, but for them food is such an emotive matter that they may find it difficult to deny food to a dog which craves it, even if this is in the dog's best interest. As when attempting to modify other owner attitudes, condemnation is counter-productive. It is much better to show some understanding of the owner's predicament. In addition, the following concrete suggestions may be helpful:

   i.   **As long as the total calorie intake is correct, food may be offered as often as before,** including tit-bits. Low calorie foods, such as vegetables, may be offered ad lib.

   ii.   Although expensive, **commercial diet dog foods** can be useful, because they are precisely measured; there is no temptation to offer 'a little bit more'.

   iii.   **Frequent weighing** by both owner and veterinary surgeon can provide rewarding feedback for the owner, as well as an index of progress.

   iv.   The owner should be encouraged to **exercise** the dog appropriately. As well as making a contribution to weight reduction, this will give the owner an opportunity to observe its beneficial effects in terms of increased fitness.

As well as being valid in themselves, these and other measures may have the paradoxical benefit for some owners of **making the process of weight-reduction complex and troublesome.** To tell an owner merely to give his dog less to eat may sound like an instruction to neglect it. To prescribe a more complex regime of weight reduction is to encourage an owner to express his affection for his dog in a more constructive way than stuffing it with food.

11.4. INAPPROPRIATE URINATION AND DEFAECATION

In the absence of physical causes, the following factors may give rise to this behaviour:

a.   **Submissive urination**

   Urination may occur as part of a response of passive submission (see Chapter 4.6) where the dog rolls onto its back with one hind leg raised (see Figure 3, Chapter 4). It occurs when an already submissive dog is approached by a person or dog it perceives as especially dominant; such behaviour is particularly common in puppies. The problem should be treated by reducing the apparent dominance of the other dog or person. For example, a person who elicits submissive urination should not stand over the dog but should greet it while crouching down to its level. He should not stretch out his hand above the dog but allow it to approach him; he should also slightly avert his gaze and not look directly at the dog. Engaging it in play may help. If the behaviour is provoked by another dog, that dog should only be allowed to meet it under restraint or supervision, until it becomes more confident.

b. **Stress or excitement**

Some dogs may urinate or defaecate involuntarily in response to stress or excitement. Fear may provoke this reaction, but it may also occur when visitors arrive or when the owner returns home. This kind of behaviour is also much commoner in puppies and in many cases will resolve with maturity. Meanwhile, ensuring that the dog has urinated before the visitors arrive or arranging that it greets the visitors in the garden may help. If it is troublesome or persistent, systematic desensitization to the triggering stimulus should be employed. Punishment should never be used, as it will tend to make the problem worse.

c. **Faulty learning**

Dogs may urinate (or more rarely, defaecate) regularly in the house in certain places, because they have never learnt not to. Once a scent mark has been left in a certain location, that scent will tend to trigger an instinctive response of urination again. Urination and defaecation are also subject to classical conditioning, so that, even in the absence of a scent mark, stimuli which have previously been associated with these responses tend to re-evoke them. This is the mechanism which enables an owner to house-train a dog but it is also responsible for the formation of undesirable habits.

Inappropriate urination (or defaecation) usually occurs when the owner is not present. It may seem that the problem is that the owner has not been able to catch the dog in the act and administer effective punishment. (It should go without saying that punishment some time after urination is never effective). However, the problem usually originates a stage further back. The owner has often caught the dog urinating in other undesirable places and punished it; the dog has thereby learnt to inhibit urination in the owner's presence. The result is that the dog does not urinate when the owner takes it outside, but when they return to the house it slips away into another room and urinates there.

The treatment for this kind of problem is essentially the same procedure which should be employed in house-training a puppy. The following points should be borne in mind:

i. The aim of the procedure is not to teach the dog a '**rule** of behaviour ' (see Chapter 2.5) but to build up the **habit** of urinating and defaecating in the desired place.

ii. This is done by running the dog's life so that it deposits its urine and faeces only in the desired place and therefore its scent marks are to be found only in that place.

iii. The dog should be taken out during the day when urination or defaecation seems likely (i.e. after food, after sleep or when it sniffs the ground for scent marks).

iv. The dog should preferably be taken out to a place where it can run about, as exercise facilitates defaecation in particular.

v. Owners should be encouraged to observe their dogs' behaviour closely, as impending urination or defaecation can often be predicted. In addition, this behaviour often follows a regular daily pattern.

vi. Scent marks in undesirable places should be eliminated as far as possible, using diluted bleach, a biological detergent or proprietary odour eliminator.

vii. When the dog is left unsupervised it should be made impossible for it to urinate in an undesirable place. Its instinctive revulsion against fouling its own bed can be built on by accustoming it to a be in a cage and then confining it there when unsupervised. The dog should be left in the cage for short periods only, at least initially, to ensure that it does not become distressed and that it does not foul the cage; if it once fouls the cage, it will be more likely to do so again in the future. The time the dog is left in the cage can be gradually lengthened, probably for an adult dog for 2-3 hours during the day or overnight.

viii. While this training is going on, the dog should be allowed access to the undesirable places, where it previously urinated, only under strict supervision. If it shows signs of intending to urinate there again (e.g. by sniffing), it should be distracted and taken outside.

ix. If inappropriate defaecation is the problem a change of diet may be helpful. A decrease in frequency of passing stools may be achieved by reducing the fibre content.

It is sometimes difficult to persuade owners to adopt this regime, because it may sound too much like what they have been doing already, with the morally satisfying part of punishing the dog denied them. It may be necessary to emphasise that the treatment of this problem is a time-consuming and painstaking business, but that in the end it will succeed. It may also be necessary to persuade the owner that moral concepts are inapplicable. Owners who are prepared to be tolerant with a puppy which makes mistakes in house-training may be filled with indignation if their adult dog shows similar lapses. Unfortunately, some owners with badly house-trained adult dogs have acquired these dogs as adults because they find the process of house-training tedious or distasteful. If these adult dogs have been previously kept in kennels or have had a disturbed early life, however, they may present house-training problems which are more severe than those presented by the normal puppy.

d. **Territorial marking**

Urination (or more rarely defaecation) may be used as a social signal for marking territory. When it fulfills this function, small amounts of urine may be deposited relatively frequently. There may be no obvious stimulus, but it is often done in response to a strange dog or even human visitor in the house. It may be worse during a time of stress or turmoil in the household. Male dogs are more likely to engage in territorial marking, but bitches may do it also.

Castration produces some improvement in territorial urination in 50% of male dogs (Hopkins, 1976). It is advisable, first of all, to test the likely effect of castration with delmadinone. If this is ineffective, or in the case of castrated males or bitches, megestrol should be tried. In some cases, the frequency of territory marking may be connected to a high dominance status. Where this seems to be the case, the dog's dominance should be reduced.

As regards behavioural treatment, close study of the dog's behaviour may reveal the stimuli triggering the urination. Thus, it may occur when visitors arrive or when the dog is allowed in a room it does not often visit. The dog should be kept under supervision when the stimuli occur. If it shows signs of intending to urinate it should be prevented or distracted and a reward given for an alternative response. The urine marks should, of course, be thoroughly cleaned.

Urination or defaecation in the owner's absence is often just one aspect of restless or destructive behaviour due to agitation at being separated from the owner. Where this is the case, the underlying agitation must be treated (see Chapter 10.6) before the problem will resolve. Even where no other signs of agitation are evident, where the urination or defaecation occur only when the dog cannot reach the owner, separation anxiety must be considered as a possible causal factor. In many cases, it is probable that faulty learning also occurs; once the dog develops the habit of urinating in a certain place when on its own, it is more likely to continue. When the separation anxiety has been treated, confining the dog in another room, where urination has not previously occurred, may solve the problem.

Urination or defaecation during the night. In the absence of physical abnormality, an adult dog should last through the night without needing to urinate or defaecate. Before proceeding to more elaborate measures, it is worth checking that (a) the dog is taken out to urinate last thing at night or defaecates outside sometime following its evening meal and (b) no food or water is given for two hours before it is taken out or left out at night.

Urination or defaecation which persists in the face of these measures is often another form of separation reaction, the dog becoming agitated when shut away from the owner for the night. Where this is the case, the problem is easily solved by allowing the dog access to the bedroom. Where the owner will not contemplate this solution, an alternative is to get up during the night and let the dog out before it urinates. This presupposes that the owner has first determined the time during the night when the urination occurs. When this regime is successfully established, the dog is gradually let out later and later.

In some cases the dog urinates or defaecates at night, even when it has free access to the owners. This is likely to be due to faulty learning. One way of retraining the dog is for the owner to make sure that he wakes and takes the dog out before it urinates. This might be done by settling the dog beside the bed and putting it on a lead with the other end around his own wrist so that when the dog wakes and starts to wander around looking for a place to urinate, the owner will be woken. He should make the dog lie down again and, when it is calm, take it outside to urinate. On subsequent occasions the lengths of time the dog is required to wait should be gradually extended until eventually the dog lasts the night. Once this regime is under way, it may not be necessary for the owner to be physically attached to the dog; it may well come and wake him up when it needs to urinate.

11.5 INAPPROPRIATE SEXUAL MOUNTING

This may consist of mounting inanimate objects, such as rugs, pillows or soft toys or it may consist of mounting people, usually children or visitors. This kind of behaviour is common in puppies, but may persist into adulthood in a few dogs. It is normally shown by male dogs, but bitches may also do it, especially before or during oestrus.

CAUSES

Although hormonal factors obviously influence the behaviour, it often seems to be less an expression of bizarre sexual preference than a displacement activity in response to conflict or excitement (see Chapter 5.4). Thus, visitors are common targets because of the conflicts between friendliness and aggression which they may arouse. Similarly, children are apt to behave in a more excitable way with dogs, giving them contradictory signals which they find hard to interpret. A dog may learn to associate this kind of interaction with children, so that a child who is mounted may not himself have behaved in this kind of way towards the dog, but may be the victim of the dog's past experience. Similarly, an inanimate object which at first was used as a target for displacement activities just because it happened to be handy, may subsequently take on a special meaning to the dog. Sexual arousal is subject to classical conditioning, so that once a dog has come to associate sexual arousal with a particular object, however inappropriate, this association is liable to persist unless active steps are taken to discourage it.

TREATMENT

An appropriate combination of the following methods may be tried:

a.   Castration produces some improvement in 60% of male dogs which engage in the behaviour (Hopkins, 1976). Its probable effect should first be tested with delmadinone.

b.   In bitches or castrated male dogs, megestrol may be effective. Castration or treatment with synthetic progestagens should always be accompanied by behavioural methods of treatment.

c.   If the target is a particular inanimate object, it may be possible temporarily to put it where the dog cannot reach it. The dog should then be gradually allowed access to it, under supervision.

d.   The owner should carefully observe the situations in which the mounting occurs. If these seem to include features which might be inducing conflict in the dog, steps should be taken to reduce that conflict. For example, visitors might be instructed not to greet the dog or children might be shown how to play with it gently.

e.   In situations where the mounting is likely to occur, the dog should be kept under close supervision, preferably on a lead. If it shows signs of intending to mount, it should be distracted and an alternative response substituted.

11.6. UNCONTROLLABLE BEHAVIOUR ON WALKS

For many people, one of the great pleasures of owning a dog is the shared enjoyment of walks together. For some, however, this pleasure is marred by various irritating features of the dog's behaviour. Two of the most common are:

a. **Not coming when called.** Judging by the number of owners who can be seen in public parks vainly and desperately calling their dogs' names, this tendency must be widespread. Investigation usually reveals that one or more of the following factors is operating:

   i. **The dog may be engaged in an instinctive response so strong that it overrides the learned response of coming when called.** Examples of such instinctive responses are chasing prey and following bitches in oestrus.

   ii. **Analysis of the interaction between dog and owner may reveal that the owner is inadvertently rewarding the response of not coming and punishing the response of coming.** Most owners realise that hitting or shouting at the dog when they finally get hold of it is counter-productive, but many speak softly and enticingly to the dog when it hovers at a distance, but grab at it when it comes within reach. The owner should take care only to pay attention to the dog as long as it continues to approach him. When it actually comes to hand, he should supplement the praise with tit-bits. Only after the dog has been rewarded should it be taken hold of and put on the lead. If the dog hesitates in its approach to the owner, the owner should immediately ignore it, perhaps even turning his back.

   iii. **Often dogs which do not respond when called have learnt to associate their names with the act of running away.** Every time the owner vainly calls its name as it disappears into the distance, this association is reinforced. To reverse this association, the owner should for the time being cease to use the dog's name as a command, but rather as a description of a situation; thus, he should frequently call the dog's name when he sees it approaching him, never when he sees it running away. The next step is to use the name as a command only in situations when the dog is virtually certain to obey (e.g. at meal times). The range of situations in which the name is used as a command should then be gradually extended.

   iv. **To some extent, whether a dog comes when called or not, may be an issue of dominance.** If it is showing signs of becoming dominant in other situations, it may be helpful for the owner to improve his own dominance generally (see Chapter 9.8). In the particular situation of trying to retrieve the dog on a walk, the owner should take care never to chase or to follow the dog because this puts him in the subordinate position, with the dog as leader. If the owner ignores the dog and assumes it will follow, he is then in the dominant role. This might seem a recipe for completely losing the dog but dogs which are not under the influence of some overwhelming instinctual drive, as in (i.), but are just refusing to come to hand, are normally careful to keep the owner in sight. If the owner walks away they usually follow. The owner should experiment with various possible ruses for inducing the dog actually to come up to him. Leaving the park where they have been walking or getting into the car usually succeeds, but this may put the dog at risk from traffic. Other possible stratagems are sitting or lying down, producing something to eat or paying attention to another person or dog. These procedures can then be phased out as the habit of following the owner is established.

b. **Pulling on the lead.** This may be part of a general picture of excitable behaviour or it may be an isolated problem. Analysis of the situation usually reveals that the pulling is being rewarded by the walk continuing and therefore by new and interesting sights and smells. This situation can be reversed by the owner turning round and retracing his steps immediately the dog starts to pull. The turning round should be preceded by a command such as 'Heel' so that eventually the command alone will be enough to stop the pulling.

Choke chains are not normally useful as the sensation of being pulled at the neck instinctively makes the dog pull in the opposite direction. Head collars (see appendix), which fit over the dog's head and allow it to be controlled in the same way as a horse is led, may prove useful in some cases.

FURTHER READING

VOITH, V. L. and BORCHELT, P. L. (1985). Elimination behaviour and related problems in dogs. Compendium on Continuing Education for the Practicing Veterinarian, 7, 537-544.

MCKEOWN, D., LUESCHER, A. and MACHUM, M. (1988). Coprophagia: Food for thought. *Can. Vet. J.* **28**, 849-850.

PREVENTION OF BEHAVIOUR PROBLEMS

Chapter Twelve

**Breeders' responsibility; selecting a breed; deciding on sex of dog;
where to buy a puppy; where to buy an adult dog;
acquiring a second dog; choosing a puppy; rearing a young puppy;
separation; house-training; undesirable behaviour;
specific problems; later training.**

It is much easier to say how, in an ideal world, most dog behaviour problems could be prevented than to put such recommendations into practice. However, as a profession, veterinary surgeons are the best placed to disseminate information and bring pressure to bear on the two groups of people who have the most influence on the development of behaviour problems: breeders and owners.

12.1. BREEDERS' RESPONSIBILITY

Genetic factors

There is no doubt that there are genetic factors associated with most dog behaviour problems. Breeders therefore have a responsibility to discard from their breeding programmes any dog of unsound temperament. There is often a great temptation not to do so, as such defects may not be obvious in the show ring in the same way as defects of conformation. It would be possible to devise screening tests along the lines of those already employed for physical defects. Many milder behavioural defects which are only manifested in the presence of specific stimuli would slip through the net, but it should be possible to detect more marked cases of dominance aggression, excitability and fearfulness. **The importance of eliminating genetic predispositions to behavioural problems should not be minimised. It is arguable that behavioural problems cause more long-term misery to owners than almost any physical defect.**

Early environment

Given the evidence regarding the crucial psychological importance of a puppy's social and physical environment from 3—12 weeks of age (Chapter 6.2), breeders have a responsibility to rear their puppies in an environment which provides constant human contact and exposure to domestic sights and sounds.

Choosing owners

Breeders also have a responsibility to match to some extent the likely future temperament of the puppies they are selling with the experience, personality and life-style of the owners. For example, breeders of working dogs, such as Border collies, should try to ensure that a prospective owner intends to train the dog and keep it adequately occupied; breeders of large dogs prone to dominance aggression, such as Rottweilers, should ensure that the owner is capable of controlling it adequately. It is arguable that breeders of such specialist working breeds should not sell them as pets.

HOW OWNERS CAN PREVENT BEHAVIOUR PROBLEMS

It is, perhaps, the exception rather than the rule that an owner asks the advice of his veterinary surgeon before acquiring a dog. However, opportunities do arise for offering such advice, which may well be of a kind which the owner can obtain nowhere else.

12.2. SELECTING A BREED

Although the temperament of a pedigree dog cannot be predicted as accurately as its physical appearance, each breed carries a raised probability of the appearance of certain behavioural traits and a decreased probability of others. Many owners do not seem to appreciate this and select a dog on the basis of physical appearance alone. Others may generalise from a sample of one and buy the same breed as, say, a friend's dog they have known and liked. Even the more careful owners who try to find out more about the temperament of various breeds may have difficulty in doing so. A book on the subject of a particular breed of dog is usually written by someone who breeds them and tends to be heavily biased in their favour; furthermore, the breeder may also be so experienced in dealing with his particular breed that he may not be aware of the difficulties which some of its characteristic behavioural tendencies may pose for the ordinary pet owner. In addition, many handbooks which survey all the breeds of dogs commonly available use the kind of language which bears the same relationship to reality as an estate agent's description does to an actual house. For example for 'independent-minded' or 'good watch-dog' read 'inclined to dominance aggression'.

In terms of personal advice, the veterinary practitioner is one of the few people from whom the owner can get unbiased advice in choosing a dog. As well as the more obvious parameters (size of house and garden, time available for exercise and grooming etc.) the prospective owner should be encouraged to consider his own personality and what emotional needs he wants the dog to satisfy. The veterinary practitioner should help him to see what kind of relationship is likely to develop between him and a particular type of dog. If the dog is to live in a family, they should be helped to consider what impact that household is likely to have on the dog. For example, a single woman who wants a close emotional relationship with her dog should not have a male dog of a breed inclined to be dominant; a family with young children where there is inevitably quarrelling and a good deal of excitement should not get a dog of a breed inclined to anxiety or hyperactivity.

Most small animal veterinary practitioners see enough dogs to be able to form an opinion as to the behavioural characteristics of various breeds. Even so, the findings of a survey carried out by Hart (1983) of the opinions of a large group of American veterinarians and obedience judges may be of interest. They were asked to rate 56 breeds on 13 personality traits. Cluster analysis showed that these traits could be grouped into three general characteristics: reactivity (i.e. excitability or hyperactivity) aggressiveness and trainability. Breeds considered to be prone to high reactivity included cocker spaniels, Yorkshire terriers, poodles, Shetland sheepdogs and pekingese. Those considered to be prone to aggression included Alsatians and Rottweilers. Those considered to be prone to both included chihuahuas, Scottish cairn and West Highland white terriers. Breeds low in both reactivity and aggression included Labradors and golden retrievers.

One of the drawbacks of this kind of study, however, is that it does not take account of regional variations. For practical application, its findings need to be modified in the light of local knowledge.

12.3. DECIDING ON SEX OF DOG

Owners are often less willing to acquire a bitch because of the risk of unwanted pregnancies. There is no doubt, however, that dogs are much more likely than bitches to develop behavioural problems such as territory marking, roaming, mounting and various forms of dominance aggression (Voith & Borchelt, 1982). Moreover, castration neither prevents nor can be relied on to treat such disorders (Hart & Hart, 1985). Owners who are undecided about the choice of sex should be advised to choose a bitch and take appropriate steps to avoid pregnancy.

12.4. WHERE TO BUY A PUPPY

Owners who want a puppy should be urged to buy one direct from the breeder rather than to buy one which has had one or more intermediate homes. Apart from the unsettling effect which changes of environment are bound to have, buying from a source which is not the breeder makes finding out about the puppy's background and early life much more difficult. Commercial dealers, including pet shops, are particularly to be avoided, because the puppies usually have so little social contact with people and such a limited physical environment.

When buying from a breeder, the owner should satisfy himself that the puppies have been kept in optimum conditions for socialisation from the age of three weeks, i.e. that they have been kept in the house, with plenty of contact with litter-mates, mother and people.

The optiumum age for puppies to go to a new home is one at which the puppy is sufficiently mature to leave its mother and litter mates but which also maximises the puppy's opportunity for early experience with dogs, people and everyday sights and sounds (see Chapter 6.2). The optimum age, therefore, depends on the circumstances of the individual breeder and owner, but 8 weeks seems satisfactory in most cases.

Serious dog breeders often disparage owners who dabble in breeding, allowing their pet bitches to have one or two litters. The grounds for this condemnation are presumably that the resulting puppies are less likely to be promising show specimens. Also, the delivery and rearing of the puppies is likely to proceed more smoothly for experienced owners and dams. From the point of view of the prospective owner, however, there is much to be said for purchasing a puppy from an amateur breeder. The amateur breeder is less likely to rear puppies in a kennel separate from the household; the event is more likely to be special for the whole household and puppies more likely to spend their important early weeks in the bosom of the family, receiving individual attention.

12.5. WHERE TO BUY AN ADULT DOG

Some owners want to acquire a dog as an adult or older puppy. The usual motive for this is to avoid the behavioural problems such as lack of house-training, hyperactivity and destructiveness which normally accompany puppy-hood. In order to succeed in this, however, great care must be taken in the choice of a dog. Many adult dogs which change owners have behavioural problems which are much more difficult to eradicate than if they were puppies. A raised incidence of behavioural problems is to be expected in dogs obtained from an animal shelter which admits dogs indiscriminately. In such a group are bound to be over-represented (a) dogs which have been rejected because of behavioural problems (b) dogs which are prone to roaming (c) dogs whose previous owners have neglected or maltreated them. In particular, it has been found that destructiveness in the owner's absence is more common in rescue dogs (see Chapter 10.7). Owners should also be cautious about dogs discarded by breeders as adults. If these dogs have not lived as house pets, they may not be sufficiently house-trained or may lack basic obedience training.

The most satisfactory way of obtaining an adult dog is usually directly from its previous owner, who can then be questioned about its previous history and reasons for parting with it. Advertisements in local papers are a good source of such dogs and many breed societies act as clearing houses for transactions of this kind. There are also some animal shelters which screen their admissions with great care and attempt to match dog to owner. Recently, the need has been highlighted for permanent or foster homes for pets belonging to elderly people who have to go into residential care or sheltered housing where pets are not permitted or who become unable, either or temporarily or permanently, to look after their pets. There are organisations (see Appendix) which put potential foster or adoptive owners in touch with such people. Some owners find a special satisfaction in taking on a dog which would otherwise be homeless and ultimately destroyed. These two latter alternatives offer the chance to be charitable in this way with much reduced risk of behavioural problems.

12.6 ACQUIRING A SECOND DOG

Acquiring a second dog is not something to be undertaken lightly. For most dogs, interacting with another dog in the household is an important part of their lives and it is a part which is difficult for an owner to control or manipulate. Another dog is a cure for few behaviour problems and may make many worse. Excitable behaviour, such as barking, may gain a whole new set of rewards in the excited responses of the other dog. Dominance problems can be harder to cure because the dominant dog has a subordinate in the family in the shape of the other dog.

If the owner has decided to have two dogs, the risk of problems will be reduced if the following conditions are observed:

a.   If the second dog is acquired as a puppy, the owner should spend extra time interacting with it on a one-to-one basis, to prevent it from forming a stronger attachment to the other dog than with human beings (see Chapter 6.2).

b.   A young puppy should not be permitted to behave aggressively towards the elder dog, even in play, as this behaviour may generalise to other dogs (Rogerson, 1991).

c.   Two dogs (or two bitches) of similar size should be avoided, to reduce the risk of dominance conflict between them. A dog and a bitch is the best combination.

d.   Two puppies from the same litter are a combination especially to be avoided, both because of the risk that they will become socialised perferentially to one another and because of the risk of dominance conflict.

12.7. CHOOSING A PUPPY

As well as investigating the environment in which the puppy has spent its early life, the prospective owner should ask to meet the dam, to satisfy himself that she is not so aggressive or neurotic that she cannot be trusted in company. Of course he should also meet the puppy and observe it interacting with its litter mates.

It used to be thought that a fairly elaborate battery of tests of the kind devised by Campbell (1975) was useful in predicting the puppy's future temperament. However, it has been shown by Young (1986) that these have poor predictive value. Certainly at 6 to 8 weeks there is no stable dominance hierarchy within most litters (Bradshaw and Nott, 1992). On the other hand, it would be silly to ignore such obvious warning signs as a puppy which growls or bites when picked up or restrained. Fearfulness can be more reliably predicted at 8 weeks (Goddard and Beilharz, 1986) and it would be sensible to avoid a puppy which seems nervous or withdrawn.

12.8. REARING A YOUNG PUPPY

If veterinary surgeons comparatively rarely have the chance to advise owners before they get their puppies, they usually have a golden opportunity just after the puppy has been acquired, when it is brought to be vaccinated. Many potentially problematic situations can be identified at this stage, where the owner is, for example, inexperienced, inappropriately moralistic about the puppy's behaviour or over-concerned; or where the puppy is nervous, excitable or aggressive.

Owners should be prepared to devote a good deal of time to their puppies, at least during the socialisation period. Many people who have not owned dogs before do not expect a puppy to be so demanding or time-consuming. Formal training which needs self-control on the puppy's part, such as walking to heel or sitting and staying, is not a priority; this instrumental learning can take place at any time. What is important is the quality and quantity of social and environmental experience the puppy gains during this period.

There is an analogy here with human infancy. A baby is not expected to learn to become a responsible and caring member of society in the first six months of life, but a good experience of a close relationship with his mother will enable him to become one in later life. A bad relationship at this stage will considerably prejudice his chances of becoming a stable adult. In the same way, a young puppy must learn in the first twelve weeks how to interact with human beings: to take part in a 'dialogue', where each responds to the other's vocal signals and body language. In order for that learning to take place, there must be responsive human beings available, who are taking the trouble to observe and interpret the puppy's behaviour.

At this time, the puppy also needs to have breadth of social experience: to meet human beings of various kinds, including children, so that it will not behave warily or aggressively towards them in later life. It also needs an interesting and varied physical environment to develop cognitive and manipulative skills. It should be exposed to experiences such as the sight and sound of traffic and riding in a car, which might cause problems later. It is unfortunate that vaccination programmes place restrictions on where puppies can go during the socialisation period. However, with a little ingenuity, many of these restrictions can be circumvented. A puppy can go for car rides without going out in the street and it can be carried in its owner's arms when she goes to post a letter.

It is also important that the puppy have social experience with other dogs, but vaccination programmes make this particularly difficult to arrange within the optimum socialisation period. In some areas, socialisation classes are held for puppies which have just completed their vacinations; these should be particularly recommended to owners of single dogs.

12.9. SEPARATION

The puppy should be acclimatised to separation from the owner. It is important that this be done on a gradual basis: young puppies should not be left alone for hours on end; on the other hand, a puppy which has never been left and then, when it is older, is suddenly faced with separation, is liable to develop separation anxiety.

The issue of dogs in bedrooms is an emotive one, on which the veterinary surgeon is well advised not to take sides if he can help it. From the point of view of behaviour problems, no general recommendation can be made. For example, a dominant dog should certainly not be allowed in the bed, but there is much to be said for allowing it to sleep on the bedroom floor. There it is in the owner's territory, but in a subordinate position; sleeping in the kitchen, it may perceive itself as being on its own territory. Night-time separation problems are usually successfully treated by allowing the dog access to the bedroom; but a dog which is accustomed to spending the night with its owner may be distressed if forced to spend a night alone.

There is much to be said for getting a puppy accustomed to being in a cage for short periods so that it is viewed as a familiar and secure den. There are many occasions in a dog's life where the ability to stay calmly in a cage is useful. To build up these positive associations, the puppy should not be confined for long periods but put there with its bed when it is about to go to sleep. Once it is asleep, the door should be opened so that the puppy can leave the cage when it wakes.

12.10. HOUSE-TRAINING

This is one specific set of responses which has to be taught early on. It can begin as soon as a puppy is observed looking for scent marks at around the age of eight weeks. The procedure is the same as that outlined in Chapter 11.4. It will be noted that, especially in the case of a puppy, which needs to urinate frequently, this procedure calls for constant attention to its behaviour. It is much more difficult to house-train a puppy which is left unsupervised for long periods.

12.11. UNDESIRABLE BEHAVIOUR

Given the opportunity, puppies will engage in a wide range of activities, some of them undesirable: they will jump on the furniture, pester for tit-bits at the table and for attention at other times, chase other animals, such as cats, jump up in greeting and so on. The best way to avoid this is to foresee these situations and run the puppy's life according to a positive routine which prevents it from being exposed to temptation. For example, chewable objects should be kept out of reach and the owner and visitors should crouch down to greet the puppy so that it does not have to jump up. When it does engage in undesirable behaviour, punishment should not be used: it should be distracted and an alternative response substituted and rewarded.

12.12. SPECIFIC PROBLEMS

Where a puppy is excessively fearful, systematic desentitisation should be carried out as described in Chapter 8.9. In addition, special attention should be paid to exposing the puppy, during the socialisation period, to as wide a variety of experiences as it can tolerate without fear. This is likely to compensate somewhat for a deficit during the early socialisation period.

Some puppies show dominant behaviour at an early age, growling, biting (not in play) guarding food, or refusing to be restrained. Sometimes, owners are unaware of the implication of this behaviour, attributing it to teething or playfulness. These cases often also show dominant behaviour in the veterinary surgeon's consulting room, and it is up to him to warn the owner of the dog's likely temperament as an adult. The owner should be encouraged to monitor all his interactions with the puppy, being careful always to maintain his own dominance as outlined in Chapter 9.8. He should also be warned that the problem may return or get worse when the dog reaches puberty and when it reaches adulthood (at about 2 years).

12.13. LATER TRAINING

Owners often ask whether they should take their dogs to obedience classes. These have the advantage that the dog meets other dogs, although most do that anyway on walks, under less artificial circumstances. They also motivate the owners to train their dogs, by providing a social setting for this. On the other hand, there may be disadvantages. Owners may be tempted to consider they have done all that is necessary to train their dogs, which is rather like expecting children to behave themselves just because they have been to Sunday School. A dog becomes a pleasant and well-behaved family member as a result of its interaction with its owners throughout the day, rather than as a result of an hour's training class. Many dogs with behavioural problems perform excellently at obedience drill. Although it is certainly desirable that the dog learns to perform certain responses on command, and such learning forms part of the treatment programme for many behavioural disorders, it is better to teach the dog at home where it is freer from distraction and is in the situation where it will eventually be required to carry out the responses. In addition, the methods used by obedience trainers vary a great deal. Some use out-dated methods, involving intimidation and punishment, which do not take into account psychological findings over the last twenty-five years. A particular class should not be recommended without some knowledge of what goes on there. When an owner can be induced to do so, it is often better for him to read a reputable book on dog training (see Further Reading) and practise regularly at home with his dog.

FURTHER READING FOR OWNERS

HART, B. and HART L. (1988). The Perfect Puppy. W. H. Freeman, Oxford.

O'FARRELL, V. (1989). Problem dog: Behaviour and Misbehaviour, Methuen, London.

ROGERSON, J. (1991). Understanding Your Dog. Popular Dogs, London.

WHITE, K. and EVANS, J. M. (1983). How to have a Well-mannered Dog. Elliot Right Way Books, Kingswood, Surrey.

GLOSSARY OF TERMS
REFERENCES
USEFUL ADDRESSES
INDEX

GLOSSARY

Behaviour therapy.

A collective term for methods, based on **learning theory,** for the treatment of psychological disorders.

Classical conditioning.

A **learning theory** term to describe the process whereby an animal learns to perform a given involuntary or reflex action in a situation which would not normally elicit it. This occurs when the natural stimulus **(unconditioned stimulus)** for the reflex response **(unconditioned response)** is repeatedly paired with a neutral stimulus **(conditioned stimulus)**. In time, the **conditioned stimulus** on its own will elicit the reflex response **(conditioned response)**.

Conditioned response, conditioned stimulus. See **classical conditioning.**

Displacement activity.

An **ethological** term to describe parts of an instinctive behaviour pattern which are performed out of context and which seem to have a tension relieving function for the animal.

Dominance hierarchy.

A hierarchical system of social interaction, seen in some animal species, in which the more senior individuals initiate and regulate more social interactions.

Ethology.

The study of instinctive behaviour patterns.

Extinction.

A **learning theory** term used to describe the process whereby an animal ceases to perform a learned response, because the response is no longer followed by **reinforcement.**

Factor analysis.

A statistical technique which enables a correlation matrix to be simplified and expressed in terms of 'factors' or dimensions.

Flooding.

A method of **behaviour therapy** for treating **phobias,** in which the patient is exposed to an extreme version of the feared stimulus, until the fear response of the autonomic nervous system is exhausted. Not recommended.

Introversion/extraversion.

A dimension of human personality, described by Eysenck, also applicable to dogs. Extraverts tend to be sociable and impulsive, whereas introverts tend to be withdrawn and cautious.

Instrumental learning

A **learning theory** term used to describe the process whereby an animal learns to perform a certain voluntary action in a given situation because that action is **reinforced** or rewarded.

GLOSSARY

Learning theory.

A collection of models, experimentally based, of how animals acquire behaviour patterns not instinctively available to them.

Neoteny.

The retention into maturity of inherited physical or behavioural characteristics normally found only in the immature animal

Neuroticism.

Used in this book to refer to a dimension of human personality described by Eysenck, also applicable to dogs (see **introversion/extraversion**). **Neurotic** individuals tend to react with excessive excitement or anxiety to outside events.

Phobia.

A persistent fear which is excessive or unreasonable.

Reinforcement.

A **learning theory** term to describe an event which is rewarding for an animal, so that if that event immediately follows an action, the probability of the animal repeating the action is increased.

Shaping.

A **learning theory** term to describe a method of teaching complex responses by **reinforcing** successive approximations to the desired response.

Socialisation period.

In dogs, this refers to the period between 3 and 12 weeks of age, when they are particularly sensitive to environmental and social experiences.

Stimulus generalisation.

A **learning theory** term to describe the phenomenon whereby a response, learned to a particular stimulus, is likely to be performed also in the presence of a similar stimulus.

Systematic desensitization.

A method of **behaviour therapy** used to treat anxiety, in which the patient is induced to perform some response incompatible with anxiety, in the presence of the feared stimulus.

Unconditioned response, unconditioned stimulus. See **classical conditioning.**

Yerkes Dodson Law.

The generalisation (experimentally established) that too high a level of motivation or arousal can have a disruptive effect on the performance of a task; the optimum level of motivation for a given task decreases as its complexity increases.

REFERENCES

ABRANTES, R. (1987). The expression of emotions in man and canid. *J. small Anim. Pract.* **28**, 1030-1036.

AGRAWAL, H. C., FOX, M. W. and HIMWICH, W. A. (1976). Neurochemical and behavioural effects of isolation rearing in the dog. *Life Sci.* **6**, 71-78.

APPLEBY, D. (1990). Good Behaviour Guide. Dog Help, Worcester.

BATESON, P. (1983). The interpretation of sensitive periods. In: *The Behaviour of Human Infants,* (eds. A. Olivario and M. Zappella), Plenum Press, New York.

BATESON, P. (1987). Imprinting as a process of competitive exclusion. In: *Imprinting and Cortical Plasticity,* (eds. R. Rauschecker and P. Marler), Wiley, New York.

BECK, A. and KATCHER, A. (1983). Between Pets and People. C. P. Putnam, New York.

BERITOFF, J. S. (1971). Vertebrate Memory, trans. J. S. Barlow. Plenum Press, New York.

BORCHELT, P.L. (1983). Aggressive behaviour of dogs kept as companion animals. *Applied Anim. Ethol.,* **10**, 45-61.

BRADSHAW. J. W. S. and NOTT, H. M. R. (1992). Social and communication behaviour in the domestic dog. In: *The Domestic Dog: Its Evolution, Behaviour and Interactions with People,* (ed. J. Serpell), Cambridge University Press.

CAMPBELL, W. (1975). Behaviour Problems in Dogs. *American Veterinary Publications,* Santa Barbara.

COOLS, A. (1981). Aspects and prospects of the concept of neurochemical and cerebral organisation of aggression. In: *The Biology of Aggression,* (eds. P. Brian and D. Batzen), Sijtloff and Noordhoff, Rockville.

DODMAN, N. J., SCHUSTER, L., and WHITE, S. D. *et. al.* (1988). The use of narcotic agonists to modify stereotypic self-licking, self-chewing and scratching behaviour in dogs. *J. Am. Vet. Med. Assoc.* **193**, 815-819.

EYSENCK, H. J. (1960). The Structure of Human Personality. Methuen, London.

EYSENCK, H. J. (1964). Crime and Personality. Routledge, Kegan Paul, London.

FÄLT and WILLSON (1979). The effect of maternal deprivation between six and ten weeks of age on the behaviour of Alsatian puppies. *Appl. Anim. Ethol.,* **5**, 299.

FOX, M. W. (1965). Olfactory imprinting: a measure of early learning in the dog. Unpublished manuscript, Galesburg State University.

FOX, M. W. and STELZNER, D. (1966). Behavioural effects of differential early experience in dogs. *Anim. Behav.* **14**, 273-281.

GODDARD, M. E. and BEILHARZ, R. G. (1986). Early prediction of adult behaviour in potential guide dogs. *Appl. Anim. Behav. Sci.* **15**, 247-260.

HARLOW, H. F., HARLOW, M. K. and HANSEN, E. W. (1963). The maternal affectional system of rhesus monkeys. In: *Maternal Behaviour in Mammals,* (ed. H. L. Rheingold), John Wiley, New York.

HART, B. L. and HART, L. A. (1985). Canine and Feline Behavioural Therapy. Lea and Febiger, Philadelphia.

HART, B. L. and LADEWIG, J. (1979). Serum testosterone of neonatal male and female dogs. *Biol. Reprod,* **21**, 289.

REFERENCES

HOPKINS, S. G., SCHUBERT, T. A. and HART, B. L. (1976). Castration of adult male dogs: Effects on roaming, aggression, urine marking and mounting. *J. Am. Vet. Med. Assoc.* **168**, 1108.

HOUPT, K. L. (1976). Animal behaviour for veterinary students. *Cornell Vet.* **66**, 72-79.

HOUPT, K. A. and WOLSKI, T. R. (1982). Domestic Animal Behaviour. Iowa State University Press.

HYDE, K. R., KURDEK, L. and LARSON, P. (1983). Relationships between pet-ownership and self-esteem, social sensitivity and interpersonal trust. *Psychol. Reports,* **52**, 110.

JOBY, R., HEMMITT, J. E. and MILLER, A. S. H. (1984). The control of undesirable behaviour in dogs using megestrol acetate. *J. small Anim. Pract.* **25**, 567-572.

LOCKWOOD, R. (1979). Dominance in wolves. In: *The Behaviour and Ecology of Wolves,* (ed. E. Klinghammer), Garland Press. New York.

LINE, S. and VOITH, V. L. (1986). Dominance aggression of dogs towards people. *Appl. Anim. Behav. Sci.* **16**, 77-83.

LORENZ, K. (1954). Man Meets Dog. Methuen, London.

MACKINTOSH, N. J. (1974). The Psychology of Animal Learning. Academic Press, London.

McCRAVE, E. A. and VOITH, V. L. (1986). Correlates of separation anxiety in the dog. Paper presented to the Delta Society International Conference, Boston.

MELZACK, R. and SCOTT, T. H. (1957). The effects of early experience on the response to pain. *J. of Comp. and Physiol. Psychol.* **50**, 155-161.

MUGFORD, R. A. (1984). Aggression in the English cocker spaniel. *Vet. Annual* **24**, 310-314.

MURPHREE, O. D., DYKMAN, R. A. and PETERS, J. E. (1967). Genetically determined abnormal behaviour in dogs; results of behavioural tests. Conditioned Reflex. **2**, 199-205.

NEVILLE, P. (1990). Do Dogs Need Shrinks? Sidgwick and Jackson, London.

PAVLOV, I. P. (1972). Conditioned Reflexes. Oxford University Press.

O'FARRELL, V. (1992). The effect of owner attitudes and personality on dog behaviour. In: *The Domestic Dog* (ed. J. Serpell), Cambridge University Press.

O'FARRELL, V. and PEACHEY, E. (1990). The behavioural effects of ovarohysterectomy on bitches. *J. small Anim. Pract.* **31**, 595-598.

ROGERSON, J. (1991). Understanding your Dog. Popular Dogs, London.

RYLE, A. and BREEN, D. (1972). Some differences in the personal constructs of neurotic and normal subjects. *Brit. J. Psychiat.* **120**, 483-9.

SCHENKEL, R. (1947). Ausdrucksstudien an Wolfen. *Behaviour.* **1**, 81-129.

SCOTT, J. P. and FULLER, J. L. (1965). Genetics and the Social Behaviour of the Dog. University of Chicago Press.

SHENGAR-KRESTOVNIKOVA, N. R. (1921). Contributions to the question of differentiation of visual stimuli and the limits of differentiation by the visual analyser of the dog. *Bull. Lesgaft. Inst. Petrograd.* **3**, 1-43.

INDEX